PHYSIOLOGY OF FAT

A Practical Guide to Reversing Obesity, Type 2
Diabetes, Hormonal Deficiencies, and Other
Maladies of the Aging Human

Dawson K. Lopez, MSN, WHNP-BC

Dedication

This book is dedicated to all the people who have struggled with obesity, type 2 diabetes, hormone deficiencies and other related health issues without getting the information and help they desperately needed.

Also, to Graciano, who supported me throughout this process and stood by silently when, at times, my frustration with technology overflowed.

Lastly, to all the people who asked questions that I couldn't answer, causing me to research even further so that I may help them and those who come after.

To all of you, thank you.

Foreword

As a practicing physician in women's health for over 30 years, I have helped countless women with their health and weight issues. Although many times rewarding, I have met mostly frustration with the ineffectiveness of diets and weight loss programs in combating obesity. Most of my motivated patients get wonderful initial results with any program, to then stall out with their weight loss long before reaching a reasonable goal weight.

Dawson finally brings to light new and logical evidence on why nearly all diets fail in the long run. We are now understanding the role of insulin in our overall health and, most importantly sustainable weight loss. We have become a society with less than ideal eating habits, resulting in an obesity epidemic, putting our children and us at high risk for type 2 diabetes and the horrific resultant health consequences.

Through daily clean fasting as Dawson's program explains, and through healthy, appropriate supplementation and hormone optimization we can be healthy, sleep better, and have more energy. Through this, we will not only enrich our lives but affect the lives of our loved ones, family and friends.

John L. Griffith M.D.

Table of Contents

Introduction

Fat. We see it, we feel it, we obsess over it, we hate it, we even eat it. But what exactly is it and why does it matter?

In locations where the majority of the world's population lives, we tend to be more concerned with those who do not have enough to eat, yet, ironically, more people die from being obese. In fact, worldwide obesity is a much bigger crisis than hunger and is the leading cause of death and disability globally. Expectations are that these rates will continue to rise, but it doesn't have to be this way.

Over the past 40 years we have been experiencing a major change in body composition, and not in a way that can be described as favorable. These changes are seen in our everyday life; in our friends, families, coworkers, neighbors, and even ourselves. Since 1975, worldwide obesity has nearly tripled, and 2016 saw more than 1.9 billion adults over the age of 18, overweight. Of those categorized as overweight, more than 650 million were documented as obese. It's not just the adults; more than 340 million children aged 5-19 are obese.

In the United States, one in ten people has diabetes, with 90-95% of those being type 2. These numbers are staggering and appear to be increasing. Not only are they increasing, but they are increasing rapidly in childhood.

Our nation's children are in a downward health spiral beginning as young as pre-school age. A 2017 report published in the New England Journal of Medicine, indicated around 208,000 people in the U.S. under the age of 20 were diagnosed with type 2 diabetes. We know the physical devastation to the patient who is diagnosed with diabetes in later life, can you imagine being diagnosed under 20 years old? How functional and intact will their body be at age 40? 60? Life expectancy is another issue; a 55-year-old male with controlled type 2 diabetes can expect to live another 13.2 -21 more years. What about the person who has been diabetic since age 9?

Greater than 25% of Americans aged 20 and older are diagnosed with insulin resistance, and more than 30% of them with insulin resistance will later develop diabetes. Those are terrifying numbers! What's even scarier is that most don't have a clue just how close they are.

The human race is changing into something we have never seen before; obese, sick, and dying. When will this madness end? It's hard to say when or how it will stop; in the meantime, obesity continues to rise along with its associated diseases. While this contains information well known (or should be) within the medical community, until the general population is educated either on their own or by the medical providers tasked with their care, obesity and diabetes will continue to climb.

Consider the elder population; 26% of seniors have type 2 diabetes. As you probably know, diabetes is linked with cardiac disease; not great when the risk of a cardiac event is already high due to age, inflammation, and low/deficient hormone levels. Seniors very often have a great deal of difficulty navigating the health care system, add to that a chronic illness that leads to the development of other chronic illnesses, and their care may be less than optimal. This, in turn, would be putting their health in jeopardy.

Issues that typically arise during the later years, such as poor eyesight, decreased mobility, loss of independence, and other age-related problems can be an even greater dilemma when compounded by diabetes related illnesses. Diabetic retinopathy, chronic kidney disease, neuropathy, amputations, and cardiac disease may reduce their independence even further.

Obesity has affected over 93 million Americans and is linked to severe health risks. Most people don't realize or grasp the negative impact on health from excess weight and obesity. Society tends to look at obesity as social issue, one that comes with brutal emotional attacks, and more recently, praise for the beauty in whatever size one is; completely disregarding health. But in reality, how beautiful is sick or dead?

Another important question, how much is it costing for us to be this sick? The diseases associated with obesity are not limited to, but include, type 2 diabetes, cardiac disease, stroke, and some cancers. These illnesses end up costing adults more than $147 billion which is not including the cost of diabetes care. Care for diabetics more than doubles that figure on its own. Due to diabetes related illness, treatments, and disability, there is also a decrease in work productivity. This decreased productivity is a widespread problem costing $69 billion annually. Currently, the total excess costs related to adolescents alone regarding overweight and obesity is estimated to be greater than $254 billion. Worse, it's costing far too many people their limbs, eyesight, and lives. All this because of food.

Obesity and its related health issues are preventable; while many are even reversible. Unfortunately, most patients continue to be provided with outdated, inadequate information that has been repeatedly proven to be false. Studies, for decades, and in some cases over a century, do not support the mainstream methods for weight loss. Why then, many may ask, doesn't their medical provider give them appropriate ways to lose weight, to treat their diabetes and abolish the fatigue? Being a medical provider is a demanding, fast-paced job and not everyone has the time, or desire, keep current on the latest research. Without realizing they are often doing more harm than good; these practitioners fail to give their patients the medical advice so desperately needed. Instead they are recycling the antiquated, inappropriate and ineffective methods of weight loss.

The information contained in this book is not a fad diet. Many, if not most of you reading this, have plenty of personal experience with those. Along with that personal experience goes personal failure; but why is the failure rate so high? It's simple, fads simply can't change the complexity of the human body. Physiology is very straight forward; once you review and apply basic physiology, you will understand why traditional dieting doesn't work. This makes the process easier and you will see remarkable changes. Using the techniques in this book that are based on human physiology, you will be able to help your patients (or yourself) shed unhealthy pounds of fat, reverse diabetes, optimize hormones and learn other ways to become and remain healthy. Fad diets are just that; a fad that comes and goes along with the fat you're trying to get rid of permanently. They aren't sustainable but merely a quick fix that actually fixes nothing.

Consider this – your car breaks down and you take it to a mechanic. The skilled mechanic understands how it was supposed to work prior to the breakdown and knows what needs to be done to reverse the damage. If the car has an issue with fluid leaking, the smart, ethical mechanic isn't going to tell you to just put some purple goop in it to thicken it and slow the leak; that is a temporary fix and doesn't repair the actual cause of the leak. Fad diets are no different. Just as the mechanic must consider the parts and functions of the car in order to properly repair it; you must consider the physiology of the body in order to restore homeostasis.

Having been a nurse since 1985, then expanding my role as an advanced practice provider, I have had access to all the research, top lecturers at medical conferences, and the patients who trust me as I apply the science to their care. While being a medical provider in solo practice, I have more recently focused less on my specialty of gynecology, and moved forward with preventative medicine as it truly is the best medical care given.

The information in this book isn't some amazing, new revelation; it's simply me relaying to you what the studies really say, what science says, what your body, through the language of physiology, is gently reminding you to listen to. It's been here all this time; it just hasn't been thrown in our face with colorful ads, tasty shakes, and promises of success. It's not feeding the pharmaceutical companies, the costly diet/fitness industry, nor is it making headlines. It's old news with newer proof; it's time to wake up and get real, while there is still time in which to do it. This book will teach you, as a provider, how to apply physiology to prevent your patients from facing chronic illness and to reverse it if it's already present. I will teach you, as an individual, how to do the very same; you don't have to be fat or sick.

This book is designed to exist in the middle; neither too technical nor too simplistic. At times it may refer to "your patient(s)" or to "you" as it is for medical professionals as well as the general public looking for answers to their own questions regarding health and aging. May both gain insight.

PART

ONE

PART

ONE

Obesity, Type 2 Diabetes

&

Weight Loss

1

WHAT IS HAPPENING TO US?

There is no need for fiction in medicine, for the facts will

always beat anything you fancy.

Sir Arthur Conan Doyle

Millions of people around the world of all ages are struggling today with being overweight or obese. Even though we have more gyms, more health and fitness coaches, more diet guru's, and the vast quantity of information on the internet, obesity is at its highest level ever, and continues to rise. Even young children in elementary and pre-school are obese; in the United States, a study of children ages 2-19 showed approximately 20% are obese and 6% of those have extreme obesity.

Extreme obesity in children is climbing. Even though there are severe immediate and long-term health risks such as cardiovascular disease, metabolic syndrome, type 2 diabetes, and other serious health issues not typically seen in the pediatric patient, treatment options are few due to effectiveness and availability. Over the past few decades we have seen type 2 diabetes double in children and this is not projected to slow down; but actually accelerate.

Despite interventions consisting of lifestyle and behavior modification, the children have remained obese and typically regain any weight previously lost. Aside from the physical health implications, are the mental health issues that challenge the child growing up with obesity. Teasing, bullying, and isolation are not uncommon experiences for the obese child. Becoming obese as an adult has its own issues, but by the time the obese child reaches adulthood, they are already plagued with a myriad of health-related problems. These changes in weight and health are relatively new in our society which means the emotional and social issues are not something we have a history of understanding and combating effectively.

If you think about the people of the 1950s and 60s you probably do not picture them being a large, if not obese, population. They were fit, yet they were not going to gym's, were not usually doing routine workouts, and not many people were out jogging. At the same time, there wasn't the soda and refined carbohydrate consumption that is seen today. The foods were more whole and nutritious, and dessert was a treat, not something we often see as a breakfast food, snack or meal replacement. There also wasn't eating anywhere but at a table; not in the car, classrooms or desks at work. Face it; we eat (and drink) all the time! There is a reason for this, and we will get to it a bit later on.

Today, the average American woman weighs 166 pounds. The average weight in 1960 was 166 pounds – for men. Many things have changed from 1960 until today, with food and obesity being at the top of the list. Food changed, and obesity happened, along with that came an increase in disease. As smart as our scientists are, one would think they would have figured out long ago why this is happening. The fact is, they did. Moreover, it has everything to do with the natural physiology of the body and how "progress" has altered it. Yes, medical research shows how and why people got fat, but that information is largely ignored by the medical community, the food industry, and the government. Someone has a grand hypothesis and the medical community is inundated with "facts" that don't exist. These "facts" are still being inserted into medical care and nutrition advice today, to the point that it's killing our population in ways never expected. The explosion of type 2 diabetics wasn't predicted and isn't slowing. It should have been predicted and prevented; but even with now knowing the cause not only are we not preventing it but we aren't treating it or curing it. This is unfair to everyone.

Even though we know what causes people to become overweight, insulin resistant and diabetic, we continue to dance around it with all kinds of theories on how to change it; yet all miss the mark. If "X" is known to cause weight gain, why do we continue to try A E I O U and sometimes Y to lose weight instead of doing the opposite of X? We know what that X truly is, but since reversing it is free and nobody profits financially, it is not brought to the table as a solution. Instead, we hear a variety of ways to shed pounds, and if you cannot, it is the fault of nobody but your own. This is a cruel game of blaming the victim. Obesity and type 2 diabetes go hand in hand, with one, often comes the other. In the United States it has been estimated that there are more people with pre-diabetes and diabetes then there are without, and the numbers are rising each year. Often people with either of these have no idea they are insulin resistant or diabetic and are headed for a train wreck. With obesity and diabetes, cardiovascular disease develops; heart attack and stroke remain the number one cause of death in the world. Going into the year 2020, this is not where we should be!

BEING FAT

Those who are overweight know what it means to be marginalized, shamed, and blamed for their fatness. Most are aware, every minute of every day, of their weight. Regardless of how they present to the world, they do not and did not choose this life. If overweight or obese, a person's value appears to decrease in society. They are looked upon as if they were "less than" and often treated as if they were. They are deemed unintelligent and weak. "You have no will power." "If you would just stop eating so much!" "You need to exercise." "Being fat is a choice." "If you wanted to lose it bad enough you would stick to a diet." "You just need portion control." If you haven't heard those from others, you may have told yourself something similar, or perhaps you thought it about someone else. How many practitioners believe their patients who say they have stuck to the diet yet cannot lose weight or even gained more? Probably not many. Those derogatory, blaming statements and others like them are not only incorrect, but also are emotionally damaging and can lead to more despair which, in turn, often results in increased consumption. These expressions placing blame for lack of fat loss could not be further from the truth! Is it any wonder that people have begun to embrace the plus size epidemic and glorify the curves that have become a symbol of beauty in some cultures regardless of the health implications? Why fight what you cannot change or, as many practitioners and others see it, what they won't change.

People aren't making these blanket statements to be cruel; they do it out of ignorance as to what causes weight gain and obesity and what it factually takes to lose the fat. They think they understand weight loss, but in reality, they are mostly clueless. When a medical practitioner dismisses a patient as non-compliant and acts as if the patient was wasting their professional time and energy, they are close to being correct. It is, however, not the practitioner's, but the patients time and energy that's being wasted on worthless, outdated, and proven to be incorrect information.

The public has been told for decades now to eat this, don't eat that, move your body, calories in versus calories out, you have to eat often to keep the fire burning, portion control, control yourself!

We heard fat is bad; food companies took out fat and because the food lost so much flavor without the fat, they replaced it with things like high fructose corn syrup. "Eat low fat and lose weight, prevent heart disease," they told us. What happened? We got fatter, and heart attacks increased. Even our government continues to tell us to eat more carbohydrates and less fat. Diet "doctors" tell us to eat more meat, eat less meat, eat low fat, eat high fat, don't eat on bread on Tuesday... One contradicts the other, how is a body supposed to know what to do?

Right or wrong, when we hear something enough, we begin to believe what is being touted as truth, especially when it's being said by a person or entity that is in a perceived position of authority. When none of it ever seems to work in the long term, we begin to wonder if anyone really has the magic answer. It can be depressing, demoralizing and demotivating to work so hard and invest so much time, energy and emotion into something that continues to fail. Would you want to climb a never-ending mountain? Shovel a pile of dirt that never gets smaller? Losing weight can be that difficult for most people and can create a host of emotional issues relating to self-esteem and worth. This affects relationships not only with one's self but also with others. It's draining. People begin to feel as if they will never overcome the unsettling mess of what has become of their body and health, and very often give up, but not usually before trying more fat loss remedies than they can count on both hands.

Millions of Americans have listened to the advice coming from their health care providers, television commercials, friends, family, books, products, and programs. They have joined gyms, quit gyms, joined diet food plans, quit diet food plans, lost weight, regained weight, lost again, regained even more, and got sicker. Despite their best efforts, the fat is not budging and, in many cases, seems to be getting worse for trying! Are they doing something wrong? Are we giving bad advice? Yes, they are because we are. Repeatedly. When our ill-informed advice does not work whose fault is it? Why the patient of course! Come on, is it really?

The medical community, the fitness conglomerate, television, and even the government have blamed overweight individuals for being unable to lose weight or to keep it off. Failing to lose weight, failing to control your appetite, failing to exhibit will power. When advising patients (friends, relatives, or neighbors) to do something and the outcome isn't as desired, blaming the failure on the patient is the standard. The fault is not on the part of the patient; it is the failure of the medical community, food companies, and even our own misguided government. You may be thinking, "But isn't the medical community the most knowledgeable when it comes to the human body?" Yes and no.

Yes, because the knowledge gained through research and evidence-based practice is there; no because most practitioners fail to read and appropriately analyze the literature. Keeping current on your own takes time and effort, not something everyone has the time or desire to do. Studies also aren't the easiest documents to interpret and are often misleading. Collectively, scientists have concluded that only reporting "relative" risk is deceptive and that "absolute" risk should be reported either on its own or in conjunction with the relative risk numbers. Other factors such as the number of study participants, comorbidities, and even other risks factors that were elevated while reducing one, such as the increased risk of diabetes while taking a cholesterol-reducing statin drug is essential to know. The reader should also be able to note which studies are flawed and may need to be disregarded. Many studies should be discounted due to flaws not readily seen until analyzed more thoroughly.

Another critical point in reviewing study outcomes is to note who the financial backer of the study is. A few meta-analyses were conducted of existing studies showing there is a systematic bias for positive outcomes if a sponsor who funds a study has a financial interest in the outcome. This should be a no-brainer, yet people continue to cite these biased studies and use them to support their argument.

Skilled research review needs to be an ongoing activity with any practitioner seeing and treating patients for any issue. If there isn't enough time to stay current, patients need to be referred to someone who can manage their care appropriately. When a practitioner does not know the most up to date information obtained through careful research (not relying on position statements of medical associations) and refers the patient to someone else, that does not mean the practitioner is incompetent in any way. Conversely, the incompetent provider is the one who fails to keep current yet treats the patient regardless. This inaction usually results in the patient receiving poor, outdated and inappropriate treatment.

There have been many, many studies done on obesity, and with this diligent research over a couple of hundred years, you would think we know weight gain and weight loss backward and forward. You would be correct, we actually do. Research has been conducted on fat gains and losses using conventional diet plans; calorie reduction, low fat, high protein, portion control, food restriction, and diet pills. While some of these things actually do work, the results are typically temporary. You can lose thirty pounds eating low fat and restricting calories, but over time this comes to a screeching halt, and you find it's no longer working or has even reversed itself. Now, even though you are still eating the same number of calories and the same foods, you aren't just not losing anymore, but you're actually gaining weight!

The truth is, it is pretty clear what causes fat gains and losses, however, information has been put out to the public for decades that directly contradicts the abundance of data we have had available to us. It's hard to change in our minds what we have had handed to us as "fact" for so long. Ingrained in the minds of Americans is that dietary fat makes you fat and raises cholesterol, which leads to heart attack and stroke. We believed that, even without a shred of evidence and a wealth of contradictory, scientific conclusions. When this false information was put out to the public there were only two studies that tested the effect of dietary fat on heart disease and they were contradictory of one another.

Something happened that completely changed the next half century on Friday, January 14th, 1977. Senator George McGovern announced new dietary goals for the citizens of the United States. He based these goals on one of the two studies, the disputed and disproven Seven Country Study, conducted by Ancel Keys. It basically put out the false information that Americans could improve health by eating less fat. Of course, now we know that is not only incorrect, but is exactly opposite of the truth. Dietary fat is essential! The only thing low fat did was increase the bottom line of food manufacturers and low-fat diet "guru's", while making us fatter. "But my doctor says…"

Most medical providers also don't know the truth behind weight gain; therefore, as previously stated, they continue to pass on incorrect information to their patients. Before you can prescribe for patients or begin a plan for fat loss for yourself, you should have a good understanding of what makes the human body gain and lose fat, and why. A weight loss plan is more effective when you understand the how and why, making it more of a conscious choice to do or not do something, versus being told what you can and cannot do without really understanding the reason.

To extrapolate what can be done to reverse fat accumulation we need to have a clear understanding of what set it in motion to begin with. In order to teach patients how and why they are gaining weight or unable to lose weight, the practitioner needs to be familiar with human physiology as it relates to foods, digestion, hormones, and the conversion of food to fat. They also would need to completely discard the old, false repertoire of dieting, calories, dietary fat, and exercise.

Conventional information relating to fatness and weight loss is so widespread and ingrained that it's often challenging (even for practitioners) to completely disregard what we believed for so long to be indisputable fact. We all suffer from a term known as "confirmation bias" which is the tendency to recall information in a way that confirms a preexisting belief or hypotheses. Our brain recalls or favors information previously heard, causing us to manipulate new information to fit the old, or to completely disregard the new information as false as we continue to favor our old, comfortable, even if incorrect, information.

For practitioners, it usually takes repeating the correct information to patient after patient before we are comfortable with this new belief. Changing our mindset and others' is difficult at best; similar to how it must have been trying to convince the people in pre-Aristotle times that the world was not flat, but round. Evolution fixed that issue; now we need to evolve as health practitioners in order to begin healing our patients, as well as ourselves.

Fat accumulation is a physiological response, so it needs a physiological reversal. But isn't our physiology the same now as it was in decades past? We didn't have an obesity epidemic prior to the 1970s, why did everything change? These are valid questions, and the answer unravels a tangled web of complex agendas. Whether you want to place all the blame on those looking for financial gains or inept, but well-meaning, professionals and government officials, there is probably room for all to be accountable.

Whether you are reading this to learn to help others or yourself there is one thing you need to do; wipe out and forget all you have heard about dieting and weight loss. Forget that you learned fatness is due to consuming too much of the wrong foods and lack of exercise. Forget that type 2 diabetes is a chronic, progressive disease. Forget all of it and make room for the not new, but perhaps forgotten, physiology of fat. Human physiology is the same whether you are young or old, rich or poor, live in the United States, Bolivia, or Africa. Let's review physiology and food to gain a new understanding of not only the human body, but how and why so many people are becoming obese and sick.

WHAT IS FAT?

Do you know what fat is and what fat does? We tend to look at fat negatively and, granted, sometimes we should. But there is more to fat than just gooey blobs making your clothes smaller and your gut bigger.

Some things associated with fat are vital for life, and some things are detrimental and can shorten the life span. Fat is more than just an adipocyte (fat cell) filled with goo; it plays an integral part in overall health as well as disease. Finding that balance between the good and bad is essential when you are helping yourself and others to have an understating of weight gain, weight loss, and the protection as well as illness associated with fatty tissue.

Fat is an inflammatory organ, yes, an organ, that secretes hormones and inflammatory substances. There are three categories of fat; essential, reserve and excess. Not all fat is created equal! Two of these categories play a vital role in maintaining health and homeostasis, and one category holds the cards in obesity and illness. We will discuss the inflammatory substances later in the chapter.

Essential fat is that which protects the organs from bruising damage and infectious disease. Wait, fat is protective against infectious disease? It sure is. The bone marrow produces T-cells, the T in t-cell signifies the thalamus where these cells are kept for future use and are a type of a white blood cell that helps to fight off infection. T-cells consist of two necessary kinds, helper and killer. Killer T-cells are like scouts, they track down harmful pathogens throughout the body and launch their attack. Helper t-cells help to orchestrate the immune system defense actions. After the scouts tackle the pathogen and learn it's DNA and how to destroy it, they retain that information and are then called memory T-cells. The next time they have a run-in with the same pathogen they can fight more proficiently, and victory is achieved earlier. The memory T-cells retreat to the fat cells and lie in wait until called upon again.

Essential fat consists of subcutaneous fat that cushions the internal organs from mild to moderate injury and provides thermal protection. The physical protection isn't throughout the entire body, and it's limited to only those with moderate fatness. Abdominal protection from a moderate amount of excess essential fat in motor vehicle accident is confirmed, although excess body fat on the lower extremities appears to worsen any injury sustained. Overall, lean people fare better in car crashes than do obese. Thermal protection has been hypothesized to be increased with more body fat, this, however, has never been proven and does seem to be significantly challenged in several studies in both humans and obese mice that show no difference in thermal protection with increased adiposity.

Intramuscular fat resides within the fibers of skeletal muscles. Small droplets of this fat are located very near the mitochondria (mitochondria convert oxygen and nutrients into chemical energy to power the cells). The fat cells are an energy supply that can be used to power the body during times of physical stress, i.e., exercise. This intramuscular fat is essential emergency fuel for the body and protects the organs from shock forces and trauma. Excess intramuscular fat is not associated with weight gain, weight loss, or weight stabilization. Age appears to be the decisive, associating factor with increased intramuscular fat. This excess fat is detrimental due to its inflammatory properties and is a factor in insulin resistance and type 2 diabetes.

The second fat category, **reserve** body fat, is stored fat throughout the body that is not essential, but naturally exists to keep the body fueled in times of famine. In times of famine, the body's reserve fat is used for fuel until the next meal. Reserve body fat is not damaging unless it becomes excessive. All bodies need reserve fat, just not a lot of it.

The third fat category, **excess** body fat, is any excess above and beyond those needed for essential function and reserve. While fat is a natural and necessary component of a healthy body, excess body fat is the culprit in being overweight, obese and sick.

HOW FAT AFFECTS THE APPETITE

Satiety is the absence of hunger between times of feeding the body and satiation is the feeling of fullness while eating. The hormones that are secreted from fat are many; however, the primary hormone affecting satiety is leptin. Leptin comes from the Greek word "lepto," meaning thin and is a protein hormone participating in the regulation of appetite and fat storage. Leptin is known as the "satiety hormone" due to its role in decreasing appetite.

It could be hypothesized that the more excess fat accumulated, the more appetite suppressing hormone is available, although that wouldn't be correct even though it almost sounds right. The brain becomes sensitized to high, prolonged leptin levels and subsequently responds with resistance. When the brain is sensitized to leptin, it's not getting the satiety and satiation signals, so there is very little satiety experienced which leads to higher consumption. In other words, your brain isn't telling the body it's had enough because it can no longer hear the leptin; just like a parent tunes out the endless shrieks of a toddler. Leptin resistance is one of the factors leading to obesity.

The inflammatory substances secreted by fat are particularly pro-inflammatory in visceral fat (excess fat accumulated around internal organs such as the liver, kidneys, pancreas, heart, and intestines). The fat excretes inflammatory cytokines which leads to chronic, low-level inflammation. This inflammation is implicated in premature cardiovascular disease, atherosclerosis, autoimmune disorders, obesity, hyperglycemia, hypertension, breast cancer, and type 2 diabetes. The closer you get to glucose intolerance, insulin resistance and diabetes, the more visceral fat you have. Increased waist size is a sign of, and reflective of, how much excess visceral fat is around the organs. Think beer belly. It can also be called bread belly, pasta belly, pizza belly, fast food belly... It's due to increased insulin and fat deposits from a diet high in refined carbohydrates. What is the only thing you have ever seen Santa eat? Yep, cookies. This is a very good predictor of disease; the higher your waist circumference, the higher your risk for disease and death. So, the takeaway from this is, the bigger your bowl full of jelly, the higher your risk of disease and death.

The inflammatory, white blood cells and hormonal molecules produced in the visceral fat, go directly to the liver. In turn, this causes the liver to release hormone disrupting substances and create inflammatory reactions. Obese men or those with increased visceral fat, have enzymes that aromatize (change) into estrone which is form of estrogen that may contribute to inflammation and cardiac disease.

Since we now recognize that it's inflammation and not cholesterol that puts the body at risk for cardiac events, we can focus on reducing inflammation through diet and reduction of visceral fat instead of robbing the body of vital cholesterol with drugs. Cholesterol will be discussed in depth in later chapters. With this knowledge of inflammation, we can also apply inflammatory reduction in treating obesity and diabetes as well as many other physical ailments such as hypertension and memory loss. Hypertension is a leading cause of cardiovascular disease and greater amounts of body fat equal higher risk for hypertension. But how does fat affect memory?

A study published in the Journal of Alzheimer's Disease in 2012 conducted by the Mayo Clinic showed a correlation between elderly people who ate a diet high in carbohydrates have almost four times the risk of being diagnosed with Mild Cognitive Impairment (MCI) which is considered a precursor to Alzheimer's disease. MCI presents with problems in memory, language, thinking and judgement. The study participants whose diets were high in healthy fat decreased their risk of cognitive impairment by 42%. That's almost half a brain! Those in the study who had the highest intake of protein from meat, chicken and fish saw their risk reduced by 21%. Incidentally, older people who consumed a low protein diet have the highest rates of frailty according to a systematic review and meta-analysis of observational studies conducted in 2018.

There is a direct correlation between increased adiposity and decreased brain function, especially in terms of memory. The hippocampus is small organ within the brain's hemispheres; each hemisphere has a hippocampus. This organ resembles a seahorse which is where its name comes from. The Greek word "hippo" for horse and "kampos" for sea monster. The small organs are part of the limbic system; the center for motivation, emotion, learning, and memory. The hippocampi play a vital role in the consolidation of information from short term memory to long term memory and the ability to navigate by way of spatial memory.

In diseases of dementia, such as Alzheimer's, the region of the brain where the hippocampi are located is the first area to experience damage. The person with such damage usually will experience disorientation and short-term memory loss in the early stages. The damage can further lead to hypoxia (lack of oxygen) to brain tissue, encephalitis, and even medial temporal lobe epilepsy. Once the area has suffered greater damage, it often results in what is known as anterograde amnesia which is the inability to form new memory.

What does this have to do with fat? The more body fat a person has the higher the insulin resistance is and decreased cognition is directly associated with insulin resistance. Insulin resistance, pre-diabetes, and diabetes all cause destruction and shrinkage to the hippocampi. The size of the hippocampi is correlated with its function; the smaller it is the lower the function. So, the fatter the body the higher the insulin resistance, ergo, the more one will experience decreased brain function.

We have reviewed the basics of fat and its purpose, so what physiological action creates the over-production of fat leading to excess fat accumulation on the body? Once we examine how hormones regulate the production and storage of fat, you will have a better understanding of how and why obesity has become epidemic and why it continues to rise.

CLINICAL PEARLS

In the patient with increased abdominal fat, no matter how healthy they appear to be, always check their HS-CRP for their level of inflammation. Prevention of cardiac related mortality in these patients should be discussed and options presented to the patient for dietary and lifestyle changes. Stop relying on cholesterol levels to be a marker for cardiac risk!

Leptin resistance reduces the brain signal to stop eating, reducing satiety. The countering hormone, ghrelin, increases during leptin resistance and creates an environment of near unsatiating hunger. Improving leptin sensitivity corrects this issue and balance is restored. This hormonal imbalance is not a "choice" but rather a medical condition and needs to be treated as such. Patient blaming is not correct, reflects poorly on you as a clinician and, frankly, it's just not cool!

2

Insulin, Sugar, and Diabesity

To find health should be the object of the doctor. Anyone can find disease.

Andrew Taylor Still

Insulin is an anabolic, peptide hormone produced by the pancreas and formed in the islets of Langerhans. Its primary function is to act as the blood glucose regulator by helping glucose enter the cells to provide cellular energy. Without insulin glucose cannot enter the cells. Glucose is vital for life and must have entry to cells to keep them alive and thriving.

When food or drink (with a few exceptions) is introduced into the body, there is an immediate pancreatic response. This response is the secretion of insulin to prepare the cells for glucose. The circulating

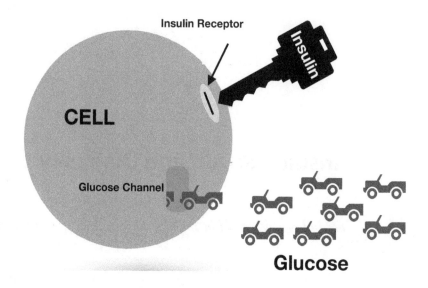

insulin acts as the key to unlock the cells and allow glucose to enter. Without glucose energizing the cells, the body will experience massive cell death which invariably leads to loss of life.

Type 1 diabetes is the diagnosis given when the pancreas does not produce enough insulin. When there is little or no production of insulin, it's like there aren't enough keys to open the locks. Glucose builds in the bloodstream (high blood sugar), and the cells are starved of vital energy. If left untreated this will lead to complete cell starvation and eventual death of the patient.

Type 2 diabetes, on the other hand, is a disease characterized by too much insulin produced secondary to insulin resistance. Just as the body can become resistant to leptin from too much stimulation, the body reacts similarly to the constant presence of insulin.

Insulin resistance isn't difficult to understand. If a person has allergies to grasses, molds or other substances what is a known treatment? Sensitization to the allergen by way of "allergy shots." This is accomplished by introducing the allergen in small enough amounts to avoid a systemic response resulting in allergic symptoms. This small amount of the allergen regularly in the body creates resistance so that the body no longer has a histamine response and the person is symptom-free. Insulin resistance works in the same way.

Imagine the cell is where the party is, glucose is the party goer and insulin are the doorkeepers. The glucose arrives, doorman knocks, the cell allows the guests entrance. But more and more guests are showing up, and the party is getting full. After a while, the doorman's knocks go unheeded. The cell is full, and it's no longer listening to the requests of the insulin. Partygoers denied entrance are building up in the hallway (think high blood sugar). Now what? The body decides the doorkeeper needs help and sends out more doorkeepers to bang on the cells, demanding the entrance of more party goers. This cycle continues as the cells become more and more resistant to the banging. But why is there a constant influx of insulin to begin with?

In years past we didn't eat as much or as often as what we do today. Once upon a time, people ate 2-3 meals per day with no (or very little) snacking. Insulin rose with the meal and fell afterward. Fast forward to 2019, and we see people feeding themselves all day. First maybe a coffee with creamer and/or sugar, perhaps a bowl of oatmeal or sugary cereal or even a cup of yogurt. Insulin rises. Before the insulin levels fall down to pre-eating levels, we may glide through a drive-thru for a specialty drink or even a diet soda. A handful of nuts or a cookie mid-morning. A few hours later it's lunchtime, then maybe an afternoon snack or drink, then dinner, then a bedtime snack or drink. That's a lot of insulin activation! This constant insulin stimulation begins, over time, to create the previously discussed resistance.

The first graphic represents how insulin levels should rise and fall with normal eating. The next one denotes what happens when we put anything in our mouths to eat or drink that causes insulin to rise. When you stop to think about the average person on an average day, we are almost constantly stimulating an insulin response. The longer the insulin stays elevated the longer it takes to have it drop back below baseline.

As you can see in the second illustration, frequent eating and drinking keep the insulin in a sustained, high mode. Fortunately, not everything, however, spikes insulin in the same way. In the Reversal chapter, we will discuss what does and doesn't have a detrimental effect on insulin levels and weight gain.

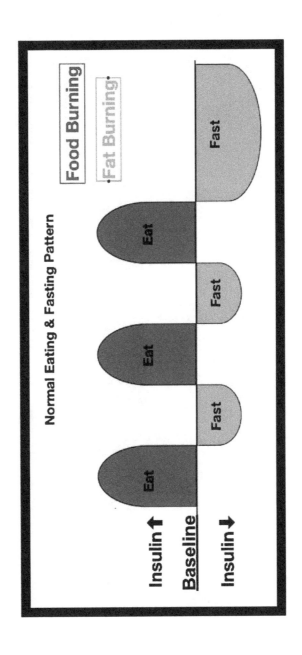

Normal Eating & Fasting Pattern

Food Burning

Fat Burning

Insulin ↑
Baseline
Insulin ↓

Eat Fast Eat Fast Eat Fast

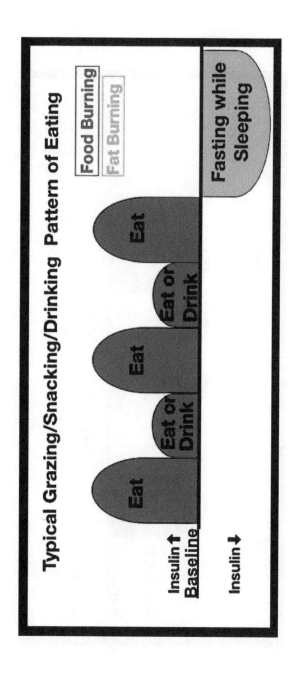

Typical Grazing/Snacking/Drinking Pattern of Eating

Food Burning
Fat Burning

Eat
Eat or Drink
Eat
Eat or Drink
Eat
Fasting while Sleeping

Insulin ↑ Baseline
Insulin ↓

44

In the 1950's there began to be concern about the possible link between sugar and cardiovascular disease. The Sugar Research Foundation (SRF) today known as the Sugar Association, embarked on a study of dietary causes of cardiovascular disease. In 1965 a top sugar industry executive named John Hickson sought to shift the concerns about sugar being a causative factor in heart disease to one that looked at sugar as guiltless. A study was launched and in 1967 the New England Journal of Medicine published a literature review which pointed to fat and cholesterol as the culprits behind this devastating health issue. This same article vastly downplayed the role of sugar in cardiovascular disease. Why would they do that?

Money. Deflection. Changing public opinion. The SRF set what the objective of the article would be, they submitted the sugar favoring articles for inclusion in the report and they received the drafts. The role of and funding from the SRF was not disclosed. The SRF paid three Harvard scientists $6,900 ($49,000 in today's currency) to publish their unfounded review of sugar, fat and heart disease. "We are well aware of your particular interest," wrote Dr. Hegsted of Harvard to the SRF, "and will cover this as well as we can."

Historical sugar industry documents suggest the SRF also funded the research that purposefully and successfully downplayed the role of sugar while promoting fat and cholesterol as the villains in heart disease. Research into heart disease was diverted for 5 decades, time wasted targeting and studying fat instead of sugar. This is a prime example of why the research done by the food industry (or stakeholders) should be viewed with skepticism. Are you angry? You should be.

Not only did the sugar industry sabotage the health of American's in the 1960's they continued with another well-known act of defiance in 2003. The World Health Organization (WHO) published a report called, "Diet, Nutrition, and the Prevention of Chronic Diseases." In it they made a very low-key statement about how it would be a good idea for people to have no more than 10% of their daily caloric intake from sugar. The went on to say that people could lower their risk of obesity, diabetes and heart disease by decreasing sugar intake.

The sugar industry was up in arms over the report and did what they could to keep that information from going public. They threatened to persuade congress to cut off WHO funding of greater than 4 million dollars per year. After a couple senators got involved the WHO decided to bury the report. The Department of Health and Human Services followed up with their own statement, "Evidence that soft drinks are associated with obesity is not compelling." Chew on that for a minute. Does it make you angry? It should.

W.F.R. Pover, from the Department of Clinical Biochemistry at the University of Birmingham in the United Kingdom, was paid by the sugar industry to do a study on sugar and its role in cancer. Of course, the sugar industry didn't want a link established and when a preliminary report was issued suggesting there was probability that the study would not be favorable to the sugar industry the study was halted on order from the sugar industry. We've all heard the theory that sugar feeds cancer, there is more to it than theory.

Three Belgian scientists conducted an almost decade long study on the relationship between cancer and sugar. Their results, published in 2017, were conclusive after being repeated three times with identical outcomes. High sugar intake by cancer cells leads to a continuous cycle of cancer growth. This process is known as the Warburg Effect which is where cancer cells rapidly break down sugars and stimulate growth. This has huge implications for cancer patients regarding the growth and multiplication of cancer cells.

If you have cancer, did your provider tell you to stop all sugar and fructose containing foods? Have you been bombarded with information on radio, television, social media, and from your medical provider about avoiding these foods? Even with the pushback from the tobacco industry, Americans were still warned in a very public way about the dangers of smoking, where are the warnings about sugar? Notably, when you go to the Sugar Industry website, sugar.org, there is nothing to be found on the study, no response at all. Crickets...

Sucrose (table sugar) is half glucose and half fructose. Sucrose is naturally occurring and can be found in that natural state in many foods, but it's added to a large variety of processed foods and beverages. Sucrose isn't a sweet as fructose (fruit sugar) but is sweeter than glucose. Sucrose has to be broken down before the human body can utilize it. The digestion of sucrose begins in the mouth where it's partially broken down into both glucose and fructose (remember, it's 50% of each) and then is further broken down in the stomach with the help of stomach acid. Sucrase, an enzyme secreted by the lining of the small intestine completes the division of sucrose into glucose and fructose. After this final cleavage the molecules of glucose and fructose can then be absorbed into the blood stream. Glucose and fructose together are a dangerous combination, we will discuss why later.

Glucose is a simple sugar, a monosaccharide. This means it's made up of one single unit and cannot be broken down into a simpler form. These units are the building blocks for carbohydrates. Glucose is often added to processed foods and you will see it listed on the label as dextrose. Glucose isn't broken down so with the help of the small intestine it goes directly to your bloodstream and quickly raises blood sugar levels. From there, with the help of insulin, it enters the cells. The juice of life! Glucose is used immediately, however, if there is an excess of glucose it is converted into glycogen and stored in the muscles and liver for future use. When called upon, it is once again broken down in to glucose and delivered to the cells.

FRUCTOSE, THE SWEET POISON

Fructose, commonly known as the fruit sugar, is also a monosaccharide like glucose and cannot be broken down into a simpler form. Like sucrose, fructose contains no essential nutrients.

In its natural form, it can be found in fruit, honey, agave, and some vegetables. While fructose is the sweetest and doesn't affect your blood sugar much, it really spikes insulin levels. Fructose is combined with corn syrup and added to foods as "high fructose corn syrup" which contains a more significant percentage of fructose than glucose. Bad news!

We've all heard this, "Fructose is natural sugar, so it's not harmful." Okay but cyanide is natural too! Natural doesn't mean free from harm, and it's naive to think the fructose in processed food has the same effects as in its natural setting within the fruit. Processing and combining fructose make this concoction a deadly recipe for disease.

Fructose and glucose are not equal and are not utilized equally in the body. While glucose can go immediately to and be used by almost every cell in the body, fructose isn't used for cellular energy and goes directly to the liver. The liver is the only organ that can metabolize fructose. So that's where goes; to be processed into glucose, lactose, and glycogen. Remember the liver can only store so much glycogen, any excess is converted rapidly into triglycerides. These triglycerides are packaged and stored in the liver and on the body as fat. This is done through a process called de novo lipogenesis which literally means "creation of new fat."

Glucose enhances the absorption of fructose and stimulates the release of insulin. With this process more of the fructose is converted to fat than would be without the presence of glucose. Eating high fructose corn syrup which is anywhere from 55% fructose up to sometimes 90% fructose, increases your triglycerides and body fat which leads to obesity and fatty liver disease, a precursor to type 2 diabetes. This is not new information! Scientists reported in 1980 that it wasn't glucose that caused insulin resistance but rather fructose. In their study, they were able to show that the participants in the fructose arm had a 25% increase in insulin sensitivity in just one week's time. That's huge. Another study almost 20 years later showed that you could take a healthy person and make them pre-diabetic in as little as eight weeks by simply adding higher amounts of fructose.

Hepatic Steatosis or Non-Alcoholic Fatty Liver (NAFL) are the medical terms for what we know of as fatty liver disease. NAFL is the result of excess consumption of fructose, usually in the form of high fructose corn syrup. Fatty liver and insulin resistance go hand in hand; it is no longer unusual to see people as young as their teens with fatty liver disease due to excess consumption of sugar-laden sodas and other foods containing large amounts of sugars. Sodas contain a very high amount of high fructose corn syrup and contribute heavily to obesity and type 2 diabetes. People who drink high fructose corn syrup containing sodas daily have an 83% higher risk of being diagnosed with type 2 diabetes over those who drink 1 or less per month.

Think about this; if you weigh 170 pounds, the sugar you consume has the cells from all 170 pounds to process ½ of it (the glucose), yet your five-pound liver gets bombarded with the other half (the fructose). That's like giving 170 people one job each and 5 people 340 jobs each. It's too much and the liver gets sick and fat laden.

Americans consumed greater than 1000% more high fructose corn syrup in 1990 than they did in 1970. A 2004 study indicated that high fructose corn syrup at that time represented more than 40% of caloric sweeteners added to foods and beverages and was the only caloric sweetener added to soft drinks in the United States. It's now 30 years past 1990, how much do you suppose consumption has increased since then? Sugar/fructose-sweetened beverages are the single largest source of added sugar intake and the top source of energy intake in the US diet.

If you haven't caught on yet, the nuts and bolts of this is that excess fructose, readily available in high quantities in almost every processed food will lead to insulin resistance, fatty liver disease, obesity, cardiovascular disease, and eventually type 2 diabetes. Except for whole foods and a few others, virtually every processed food eaten contains high fructose corn syrup. Bread, pudding, soda, candy, yogurt, salad dressing, canned fruit, frozen dinners and snacks, juice, boxed dinners, granola bars, breakfast cereal, baked goods from the store, sauces, condiments, nutrition bars, coffee creamer, energy drinks, sports drinks, jelly, and jam… so the list goes on. You probably have absolutely no real idea of how much of this disease producing product you eat on a daily basis. High fructose consumption = insulin resistance. The bottom line is that the amount of fructose consumed can be the difference between health and disease or death.

Another problem with these refined carbohydrates is that once a person eats them, they tend to crave more of them and so the cycle begins. Carbohydrates are addictive, that's why it's so hard to stop sweets, desserts, and other foods containing high fructose corn syrup after having eaten them frequently, and over time.

ANOTHER CAUSE OF HIGH INSULIN

Aside from eating and drinking there is another cause of high insulin; high cortisol. High cortisol is the result of ineffective handling of stress. Stress often comes from poor organization of time, toxic relationships, anxiety, depression, and also from not getting an adequate amount of sleep. Cortisol is a glucocorticoid (steroid hormone) produced from cholesterol in the adrenal glands. It is a necessary part of human physiology and acts in conjunction with adrenaline in the fight or flight response to situational stressors. There is a receptor on almost every cell in the body for cortisol; it plays many important roles related to function and health.

When cortisol levels rise to higher than normal levels, so does insulin. This can happen acutely with stressful situations, or chronically with ineffective coping strategies for daily, ongoing stress. Accomplishing a plan to keep stress from affecting you physically and emotionally can be a challenge and people often seek the advice of a life coach to learn how to overcome being a stress-a-holic. A life or health coach can help their client find the ways that work best for them to eliminate stressors and succeed in living a stress-free lifestyle.

Not getting adequate sleep will lead to an insulin spike that can often take a full day to lower. Your body needs at least 7-8 hours of restorative sleep per day, preferably in the night hours. Some people function best on 9 hours. If you have difficulty sleeping there could be a physiological reason behind the insomnia, or it could be environmental, or even a mental/emotional problem that needs sorted out. Have you ever noticed that after not getting enough sleep you feel hungrier than usual the following day? I've heard people say they ate to stay awake because they were so tired after little sleep the night before. They most likely ate more and were sleepier due to the increased level of insulin circulating in the body.

Low sex hormone levels can cause poor sleep in both men and women. Women often begin noticing sleep issues in their later thirties and increasing as they approach menopause with often a sharp rise after menopause. Prior to menopause this is typically due to low levels of progesterone, the calming hormone that helps you sleep. After menopause the combination of low levels of all three sex hormones can be the issue. This will be discussed in detail in the chapters dealing with hormone regulation.

When cortisol is increased chronically, there is a marked increase in abdominal fat accumulation and insulin sensitivity. Visceral fat, as previously discussed, is exceptionally pro-inflammatory giving rise to the risk of cardiac disease. Together, poor diet, chronic stress, and inadequate sleep can create a health nightmare. Add in low testosterone and low estrogen (which increases visceral fat, insulin resistance and metabolic syndrome) and you have compounded the problem. High cortisol produces an overall net acid effect which in turn leads to obesity.

PUTTING THE PIECES TOGETHER

When the body is in the fasting state, the period between eating and while sleeping, it is in fat burning mode. The body's growth hormone level is at its highest, adrenaline keeps the metabolism up, and the fat cells can be used for metabolic energy. As soon as food or drink (with a few exceptions) enter the body, the insulin spike is like flipping a switch from fat burning to food burning. This means no excess fat will be burned to fuel the body; instead, the body will be fueled by the food ingested that passes through the liver for processing.

To recap, once food is digested and passes from the intestines to the liver it is broken down with a portion being used for energy and a portion will be stored for future use, i.e., body fat. Glucose stored in the liver is converted to glycogen, but there is a limit to how much the liver will retain. Excess glucose then is converted to fat by a process called de novo lipogenesis; it's then stored in the liver or distributed as body fat. De novo lipogenesis literally means "the creation of new fat." This fat is created due to excess carbohydrate consumption which includes refined carbohydrates and sugars. These carbohydrates are converted into triglycerides and stored to capacity in the liver, adipocytes (fat cells) and released into the bloodstream. The excess triglycerides, in conjunction with an insulin resistant liver, creates what is known as non-alcoholic fatty liver disease (NAFL) or fatty liver. This creates insulin resistance within the liver and can also result in glucose overproduction and hyperglycemia.

Insulin is the root of weight gain. Have you ever had a patient or friend tell you, "I just don't understand why I'm fat (or cannot lose weight) when I don't eat very much"? I'm sure we have all heard it. The first impulse has always been one of disbelief, even inner eye rolling while thinking, "If you were eating as little as you say are, you would not be fat". Considering what was previously discussed about insulin being released all day, you can easily apply it to this situation and come to a different conclusion. With the constant influx of food and beverages passing through the body every few hours for 12-20 hours of the day, insulin is continuously high. Sustained high insulin = insulin resistance. Insulin resistance keeps the body from burning fat, leads to obesity, leads to type 2 diabetes... you get the picture. Also, Insulin effects thyroid function and thyroid function affects insulin production.

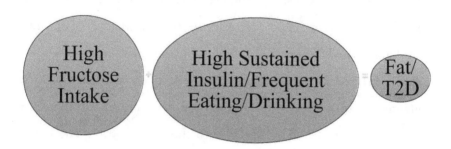

This cycle does not happen overnight; however, it can happen quickly. Most people who develop type 2 diabetes in their later years didn't start as children eating so frequently or eating the sugar-laden foods that today's diet consists of. This happened to them only in the past few decades, but when you look at the following generations, those born around 1980 and after, they started life with our "new foods" and constant eating and snacking that have only become worse as time goes on. Today's children haven't got a chance unless something is done to help them and done quickly.

The studies done with thousands of school children (and adults) to eat

less and move more proved to be major failures. Eating less and moving more did not help reverse obesity and type 2 diabetes. All of those studies of the past hundred years ended the same way — big fat failures. If you read the studies, you see the failure, yet for some reason, we still promote eating less and moving more as a weight loss plan. Does it ever work? Yes, it does, but only in the short term. It is not sustainable and eventually leads to weight regain. This eventually slows the metabolism which leads to more weight gain. There is no doubt that exercise does wonderful things in the body; improved muscle mass and strength, improved cardiovascular health, increased bone density, and decreased blood pressure. It also helps to keep depression down and optimism up. However, what it does not do is cause long term, sustainable fat loss.

Prevention is critical; it's far easier to prevent fat accumulation than it is to live with the consequences. Parent's need to be educated on how to keep their children from a life of obesity and ill health, it is a responsibility that comes with being a parent. Just as adults teach them to not play in the street or play with fire, so they are not hurt or killed, it's the parent's responsibility to raise them without making them obese and sick. It's difficult for a parent to do that when they don't know how. Our grandparents knew how to keep from getting fat and sick, but somehow their way of eating was forgotten with the advent of high fructose corn syrup, snacking all the time, and playing the blame game.

Okay, so now we understand that frequent snacking or grazing, even without consuming large quantities of food will keep insulin stimulated all day. We understand results in keeping the body in food burning and not fat burning mode. So how do we decrease the insulin, reverse obesity, reverse type 2 diabetes and fatty liver? It's not as complicated as you might think!

Understandably, it can be difficult to make drastic changes in one's life, but sometimes it can also be more comfortable than we anticipate. It seems that often the anticipation is far worse than the actual change. Keep in mind that eating refined carbohydrates and sugar cause the body to crave more of the same. When those foods are eliminated (or drastically reduced) the cravings also diminish, and it is easier to eat a healthier diet. When the results of eating a diet high in sugar and refined carbohydrates are fat gain, insulin resistance, type 2 diabetes, hyperglycemia, cardiac disease, and cancer; is the statement "but I like those foods" any reason at all to continue eating them on a regular basis? Yes, eating them on special occasions is different, as a treat, but the daily over-consumption of sugar and fructose is what needs to be eliminated. Nobody is saying you may never again have these things, but a break from them long enough to get the body back to being healthy is strongly advised.

High, sustained insulin leads to a host of problems; chronic conditions linked to the pathophysiology of insulin resistance and hyperinsulinemia: these conditions include:

- Cardiovascular disease – high insulin damages endothelial cells in the blood vessels

- Type 2 diabetes

- Hypertension

- Polycystic ovary syndrome

- Cancer (breast, colon, other) cancer cells thrive on glucose and insulin allows it to enter the cell.

- Nonalcoholic fatty liver disease (NAFLD) and non-alcoholic steato-hepatitis (NASH)

- Elevated liver function (AST/ALT) &/or GGT

- Obstructive sleep apnea

- Inflammation

- Thyroid problems – poor function and decreased T4 to T3 conversion

- Cushing's or Addison's Disease

Clinical and Laboratory Findings in Insulin Resistance

- Elevated percent body fat

- Elevated waist to hip ratio (> .85-Female, .9-Male)

- Elevated waist circumference (men > 40inch; women > 35)

- Elevated systolic and/or diastolic blood pressure (> 130/85)

- Serum triglycerides elevated (> 130)

- Serum HDL depressed (males < 40; females< 50)

- Serum triglyceride to HDL ratio (> 3:1)

- Elevated C-reactive protein (> 0.9)

- Hemoglobin A1c greater than 5.4%

- Elevated serum liver enzymes (AST/ALT or GGT)

- Elevated Apo B and reduced Apo A1

- Low vitamin D (<30)

- Damaged mitochondria which makes energy

- Elevated NMR LDL lipid particle number

- Increases kidney retention of sodium

- Decreases DHEA

- Increases sex hormone binding globulin which binds to and renders available hormone useless

- Increases synthesis of triglycerides

- Magnesium loss in urine which makes insulin resistance worse

- Increases cortisol which increases both insulin and blood glucose

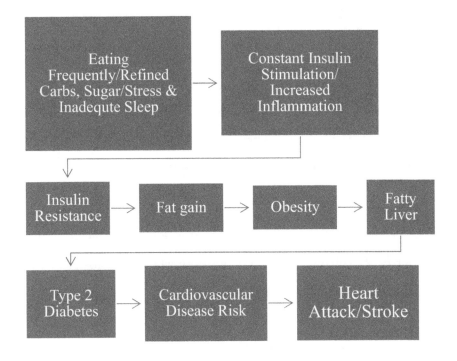

ACANTHOSIS NIGRICANS

If your patients, or you, have darker, brown to black, velvety skin on the back of the neck, forehead, armpits, navel, groin, or inner thighs, they (you) are likely to be insulin resistant. Any time acanthosis nigricans is present it needs to be investigated. I saw a patient once with what appeared to be classic acanthosis nigricans on the back of the neck yet when biopsied it was actually HPV (warts).

TYPE 2 DIABETES – THE CAUSE IN A NUTSHELL

As previously mentioned, the rate of Type 2 diabetes has skyrocketed to the point of being a severe health epidemic. It's also a money machine. The American Diabetes Association (ADA) reports that in 2017 the annual cost for diabetes care was $327 billion. Is there a more sinister reason to keep diabetes active than money? Most patients don't understand why they continue to be sick or get sicker when they are following doctor's orders. They are sticking to their ADA diet. They try to lose weight, but it keeps coming back.

Appropriate evaluations of potential causes need to be investigated. The prudent clinician will always check testosterone levels in those with type 2 diabetes, and an A1C in those with low testosterone. It is well established that men with type 2 diabetes have lower testosterone levels than non-diabetic men. This was first reported as far back as 1978, and since been confirmed by greater than twenty additional

studies — more on this in the "Andropause" chapter.

For our purpose here, we really don't need to go into more in-depth physiology of this disease when we know the underlying causes of diabetes and reversal treatment. It's more a matter of the patient receiving proper education about prevention as well as about reversal before it progresses and destroys their quality of life.

The effects of type 2 diabetes on the body can be devastating. The body is not healthy in many ways, and these out of control health issues can lead to not only a poor quality of living but kidney failure, neuropathy, loss of sight, loss of limbs, and even death. It takes a physical, emotional and financial toll on the patient and their family. And society! This is an unnecessary burden! Patients who are screened and educated early, prior to becoming diabetic, or, if the already diagnosed patient receives proper care and education this wouldn't be as much of an issue. Proper care doesn't mean giving the patient advice to follow established guidelines that are designed to keep them diabetic. Reversal is indeed possible and should be offered to every patient. If the patient chooses not to take steps to reverse their diabetes that's a choice you cannot control, however, to be an ethical provider you must still present the option. This knowledge can lead to ethical issues which won't be presented here but think about this argument; should people who refuse to take the steps necessary to reverse their diabetes be eligible for public medical assistance for diabetes related complications?

We have established that consuming high amounts of fructose can lead to insulin resistance and subsequently type 2 diabetes. Instead of being focused on lowering insulin levels, the education given to type 2 diabetics focuses on reducing blood sugar. That doesn't even make sense unless you are trying to keep someone diabetic. The excess glucose can cause problems, yes, but treating the glucose number on paper is merely treating a product of the disease and not the disease itself which invariably leads to a vicious cycle.

A very good way to monitor blood sugar levels is to not only monitor fasting levels but take a peek at post-prandial levels. Post-prandial levels are those you check about 2 hours after eating. Your blood sugar should have returned to normal. A target goal is 110, maximum. Keep in mind that being pre-diabetic with blood sugars in the pre-diabetic range is still doing damage; an increased risk of cardiovascular disease starts with blood sugars of 85. Keeping those post-prandial levels at 110 or lower is best. The insulin receptors can heal if there isn't constant exposure to insulin allowing them to function properly and let the glucose enter the cell. Once that occurs your blood sugar levels will decrease.

Labs	Optimal	Conven-tional	Insulin Resistance	Metabolic Syndrome	Diabetes
Fasting Glucose	75-85	65-99	100-119	>=100	>=120
Triglycerides	50-75	≤150	>90	>110	>150
HDL	>65	>35F, 50M	<65	<55	<55
Fasting Insulin	2-3	2-10	>3.2	>5	varies
Hemoglobin A1C	4.5 – 5%	4.5 – 5.6%	5.7-6.5%	>5.7%	>6.5 %

Regardless of your opinion as to why patients with type 2 diabetes have not been treated appropriately is irrelevant; you must do your best to rectify the situation with your patients (or yourself). If you are not comfortable dropping the current recommendations for treating type 2 diabetes and instead cure it, it is imperative that you find a provider who is and refer your patients. If you are a patient, please find a provider who has devoted the time to become educated and implement what they have learned about reversing this deadly disease. Lives depend on it. Maybe even yours. Not just for longevity but for living with a good quality of life and not one of sickness. Type 2 diabetes, when treated appropriately, is not the chronic, progressive disease you were taught that it is.

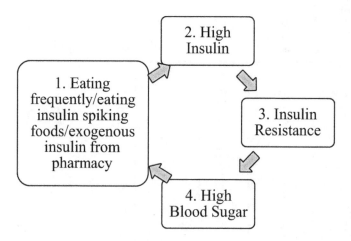

When you know what insulin does in terms of diabetes, does it make any sense at all to give patients even more insulin? Many say yes. Yes, because the oral medication is no longer controlling blood sugar. Why is that? Because they are becoming more insulin resistant because you aren't treating the disease, you're treating a resulting factor of the disease. That's one of the more significant problems with conventional diabetes management; the glycemic index. A hyperglycemic condition does not cause weight gain, insulin does. Basing the diet not on low glycemic foods but rather low insulinemic foods is the appropriate approach. Would you keep squeezing the vice tighter on the headache patient to relieve their pain? No? Yet you give the patient more insulin to shove more glucose into already packed cells which makes the patient even more insulin resistant, eventually needing higher and higher doses. Does it not make sense to treat the high insulin instead? It certainly does and is not that difficult to do. Take their head out of the vice. Give your patients three simple options:

1. Reverse diabetes, decrease risk for cardiovascular disease, live a healthy life.

2. Treat diabetes with the ADA recommendations and live with a "chronic, progressive disease," contribute to the $327 billion annual cost, increase your risk for heart disease, possibly get sicker, go blind, lose limbs, die.

3. Don't treat diabetes, definitely get sicker, lose limbs, go blind, die.

What does reversing long term, insulin dependent diabetes look like?

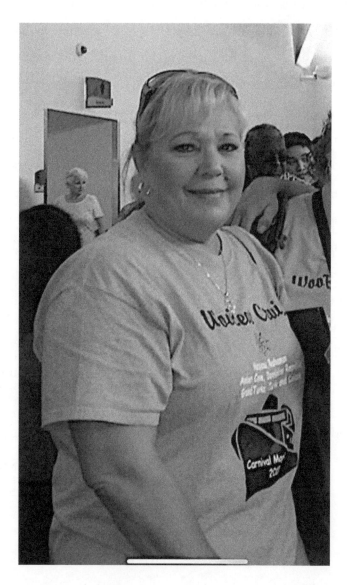

This is Paige, type 2 diabetic for 24 years, on oral diabetes medications and insulin. Desperate for an end to this nightmare she went on a ketogenic diet and started intermittent fasting.

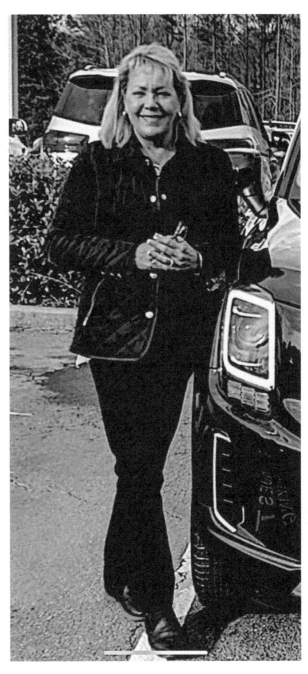

This is Paige less than a year later, beautiful and healthy!

CLINICIAL PEARLS

Disease prevention starts with knowledge; understanding that refined carbohydrates, sugar and high fructose corn syrup related disease and deaths can be easily prevented with education is the responsibility of every primary care provider. This is not necessarily nutrition counseling, rather, disease prevention. Put as much effort into teaching your patients the dangers of refined carbohydrates as you would with the dangers of smoking!

In many regions of the world, the indigenous people did not experience common health issues and "western diseases" such as appendicitis, constipation, irritable bowel, cancers, type 2 diabetes, etc. until 10-20 years after adopting a western diet that included flour and sugar. This has been well documented, as with the Pima Indians. In the 1800's they were smaller, described as "spritely" people After flour and sugar was introduced into their diet that has all changed and they now have the highest rate of type 2 diabetes in the world.

Remember to check fasting insulin levels prior to implementing a diet plan, lifestyle change, or reversal of type 2 diabetes. You will also want to recheck it periodically to monitor progress.

An average fasting insulin in the United States is 8.8 microIU/mL for men and 8.4 microIU/mL for women. People with levels of 9 microIU/mL have been correctly identified as pre-diabetic 80% of the time.

You want the fasting insulin level to be below 5 microIU/mL and ideally, at around 2.5. Over 5 demonstrates insulin resistance.

The Most Important Lab Tests for Insulin Resistance

- HgA1c
- Fasting Insulin
- Fasting Glucose
- Triglycerides
- HDL
- Post-prandial Glucose levels (multiple)

3

REVERSING THE PROCESS

"The aim of medicine is to prevent disease and prolong

life, the ideal of medicine is to eliminate the need of a physician"

WILLIAM JAMES MAYO

The funny thing about weight loss, lowering insulin levels, and reversing type 2 diabetes is it's all very similar and in most instances is accomplished with exactly the same treatment. As you have read about the physiological causes of these things you see that they are the same so you could deduce that the treatment would be the same. And you would be correct! If new food and new eating patterns made us fat and sick, wouldn't it make perfect sense to stop the new food and all the constant feeding to reverse it? Sure does. If type two diabetes and obesity is caused by X does it make any sense to try ABCDEFGNH and Q to reverse it? No, it makes more sense to reverse X.

To achieve sustainable weight loss, you need to look no further than the physiology of the human body. In order to lose weight, you need to lower high, sustained insulin levels that are keeping the body in a constant food burning mode. In order to reverse diabetes, you need to lower high, sustained insulin levels that are keeping the body increasingly more resistant to insulin. But how do you lower the high insulin?

That's where the fun begins. Remember, you must disregard any and all diet advice and food programs you have ever heard and remember the physiology we just covered. Sometimes the best way to know that you understand something is to answer the questions you have yourself. Eating raises blood sugar and insulin, sometimes just insulin, what could a person do to not raise either of those? That's right, don't eat. It's a matter of doing nothing. No special food plan to purchase, no points to count, no tasteless shakes, no pills and not shots. And it gets better, it's FREE. Not only is the whole concept free, but your food bill will be drastically reduced. WIN!

Fasting has been known to be a curative treatment for centuries. Known as the Father of Modern Medicine, Hippocrates prescribed fasting as well as apple cider vinegar for his patients a few hundred years BCE. A famous writing by Hippocrates reads, "To eat when you are sick, is to feed your illness". Plato and Aristotle were also known to support fasting. One of America's founding fathers, Benjamin Franklin, wrote, "The best of all medicines is resting and fasting". Paracelsus, the founder of toxicology wrote, "Fasting is the greatest remedy, the physician within". These men were quite smart but probably didn't realize that their words would actually be curing people of obesity and diabetes in the 21st century.

Let's look as what fasting is and is not -

- Fasting is the period of time between eating, whether it's for an hour or 63 days.

- Fasting is *not* starvation. Starvation is a state when the body has no control over when it's going to be fed and there is no longer fat for fuel.

- Fasting is *not* a fad, it's a normal part of human life since the beginning of time.

- Fasting does *not* decrease metabolism, it raises it.

- Fasting does *not* cause you to "burn muscle" when you have excess body fat.

- Fasting increases mental clarity.

- Fasting does *not* cause fatigue.

Most of us grew up hearing that if you don't eat you will go into "starvation mode" and burn muscle instead of fat. Why do you suppose that would be? Isn't the human body designed to store excess fuel as fat to use when we don't have a food source? Yes, it is. Are our bodies just confused and don't know what to use for fuel? Absolutely not. Our bodies are very detailed and intricate in their processes and work like a well-oiled machine. It will, however, burn muscle when fat stores are reduced to approximately 4%. Remember the term de novo lipogenesis? That's the creation of new fat made by the liver by converting excess glucose into fat. The liver works in wonderful ways and just as it can convert glucose into fat so can it convert fat into glucose to feed your cells. That process is called hepatic gluconeogenesis, or, the creation of new glucose. You see, your body doesn't need to breakdown muscle when it has plenty of fat to burn for cellular energy. It will, however, burn muscle when fat stores are reduced to approximately 4% as previously mentioned.

When the liver is converting fat into glucose (gluconeogenesis), over time the body becomes what we call, "fat adapted" meaning it's adapted to burning fat for fuel instead of food. By withholding food long enough for the liver to begin gluconeogenesis, the insulin level falls and the body is engaged in fat burning.

During this process adrenaline keeps the metabolic rate revved so there is no concern of slowing down your metabolism. Despite what you once believed, fasting does not slow metabolism. What *does* slow metabolism is reduced caloric intake spread throughout the day. This happens because your body is very smart and knows if too little food is coming in it must slow down body some processes that will burn it up faster, such as body temperature and heart rate. Dieters often complain of being cold and tired, the slowing of the metabolism is the cause. This is why the participants on the TV show The Biggest Loser could not keep the weight off long term; their metabolisms were trashed. With slow metabolic rates even consuming the same number of calories no longer resulted in weight loss but instead they experienced weight gain. It actually caused more weight to be regained than had been lost due to the very slow metabolism. As far as diet strategy goes, calorie restriction and exercise (together) are the biggest losers.

Unfortunately, exercise is not going to create a sustained weight loss. Exercise has so many health benefits; muscle tone, strength and density, including heart, respiratory and cardiovascular benefits, greater bone density, etc. Exercise does not create fat loss. Have you heard the saying, "Abs are made in the kitchen"? It's true. There have been multiple studies conducted for decades on calorie restriction and exercise as forms of weight loss. The results of all of them are an overwhelming failure. Michelle Obama urged schools to adopt her program, "Let's Move" while at the same time raising the amount of unhealthy carbohydrates and decreasing fat from school lunches. Again, nothing gained here except more body fat. You can't try to fix a problem with things that have been proven time and time again to not work. Okay, so exercise isn't going to reduce the fat volume, what will?

Decreasing insulin levels decreases fat. When insulin is high you may feel foggy, sluggish, or even extremely sleepy. Sometimes you don't even notice the lack of clarity, it's just daily life that you have become used to over time. Then fasting comes along and you being to see that just by skipping one meal your mental clarity is increased as is your overall energy. Your hunger is decreased and you feel great. Of course, that sounds great, so how does one go about fasting?

HOW TO FAST

I can already see the eyes rolling and hear many people groan, "I can't do that! I'll be too hungry!" There is actually no basis of truth in that. You *can* fast, but might not choose to. The hunger part is actually an interesting topic. Hunger isn't a steady thing, it's doesn't build in intensity over time, and it isn't harmful. It's more of a psychological phenomenon than a physical reality. You are no more hungry when fasting than you are when eating. It's true! Take two people, both feel hunger, one eats and hunger goes away. The other doesn't eat and hunger goes away. Please keep in mind that hunger is not an emergency! That feeling we associate with hunger is from the gut peptide hormone called ghrelin. Ghrelin stimulates growth hormone, so basically when your stomach is growling your growth hormone is high which is a great thing when trying to decrease fat. When you feel it you have a choice, you can put something in your mouth and stop the fat burning process right there and then, or you can ride it out and continue on knowing you are in fat burning mode.

I frequently hear, "I can't skip breakfast, I'm hungry in the morning. My blood sugar will drop". Blood sugar in the non-diabetic person with excess fat stores is not going to drop below normal even if you fast for 6 months. It may be lower than usual for you, but it will not go below normal as long as you have fat to burn. That's because your body is still making glucose for your cells, only now it's using your body fat instead of food.

The longest recorded fast was in a 27-year-old man and lasted for 382 days. During that time his blood sugar dropped but never below normal and all labs were stable. He began the fast at 456 pounds and ended at 180 pounds. While this type of fast is *not* something I recommend nor will I supervise, this does show that the body continues to make glucose whether it's from the food you eat or the food you have stored as fat. But what about that morning hunger?

It may have been six, eight, or even 12 hours since your last time of eating, but that's not why you are hungry. When a newborn baby comes home from the hospital and is fed every three hours it's hungry every three hours. If it's fed every four hours, like clock-work it's hungry every four hours. We set when we will be hungry by when we eat. All the time! We eat too much and too often! So, if you normally eat breakfast in the morning you will be hungry in the morning. When you stop eating breakfast you will stop being hungry for it. Hold on a minute! Isn't breakfast the most important meal of the day? We've all, undoubtedly, heard that fictional statement. Do you know where that statement came from? It wasn't science, it was a marketing campaign for breakfast food!

Typically, when you are hungry it's not low blood sugar that makes you feel off, it's often lower sodium and/or other electrolytes; have a pinch of salt or add it to your water. Not so much that it changes the flavor, just a bit. If that's a problem for you during the fasting time be sure you are getting enough electrolytes during your eating window. A great solution is to add tri-salts to your water. Tri-Salts contains nutritionally significant amounts of the essential macro minerals, calcium, sodium, and potassium, as carbonates and bicarbonates. It does not contain sodium. This can help you burn through a busy day without feeling weak or lightheaded as you fast. I would warn you against drinking much "Smart" water as it doesn't contain sodium, the more you drink the more dehydrated you become.

We all fast daily; unless you are an Ambien binge eater, we all fast during the sleeping hours. This is the beauty in fasting, most of the fasting is done while you are asleep! There are various ways to incorporate fasting into your life; it can be daily, every other day, weekly, monthly and sometimes yearly. It can be short or extended fasting. When treating obesity and type 2 diabetes, it needs to be more consistent such as daily or every other day fasting.

Fasting routines are often described as intermittent fasting due to the periods of feeding in-between fasting. Yes, this is what we already do and we are still fat, so we need to change up the feasting and fasting times. By eating your meals during a period of time during the day, called your "eating window" and by clean fasting outside of your window, the body quickly begins to lower insulin. Setting your eating window is completely individual, it can be 1 hour, it can be as high as 8 hours although that isn't the best plan for reversing obesity and diabetes. The results will vary; what works for one isn't what works best for another. Here are some examples of intermittent fasting:

Daily –

Sixteen hours of fasting and eight hours of eating time. Eight hours is a long time to have an open eating window, but for many it works quite well, especially for weight maintenance. Say you set your eating window from 12 noon to 8pm. You eat lunch and you eat dinner; you are skipping breakfast each day. You are fasting from 8pm until you eat lunch the following day, you are only missing one meal and snacks. You don't need snacks! This eating window can be as small as you choose. Many people eat one meal per day, they lose weight rapidly, reverse diabetes, look and feel fantastic thanks to autophagy which we will discuss later.

"Breakfast: the most important meal of the day!"

NO, IT'S NOT!

Marketing is brilliant but it's NOT science!

You can start with an eight-hour feeding window if you feel you need to ease into fasting, or, depending on personal need and/or preference can shorten the eating window to six hours, four hours, etc. Eight hours is actually a long eating window and you don't want to extend past eight hours. You can shorten the window by eating later in the day or by eating dinner earlier. You don't have to be exact, nor do you need to keep the same eating window each day. As long as your fasting time is no less than 16 hours it really doesn't matter when you ear. Many people stick to the same times and many change it up. Some eat during a four-hour window late afternoon through early evenings Monday through Friday and then on the weekend change it to a mid-day window.

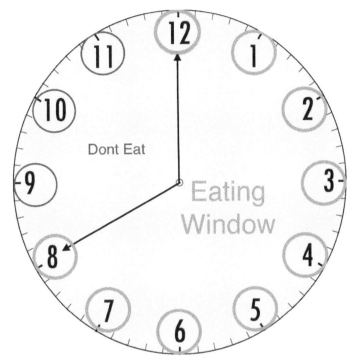

The preceding graphic is an example of an 8-hour feeding window. This doesn't mean you eat the entire 8 hours, but anything you do eat must be within that 8-hour window. Change the times of day to meet your needs; for example, you might choose 9AM to 5PM, or 10AM to 6PM.

Every Other Day and More

This can be done in multiple ways. Many people choose to eat two meals per day on day one, skip breakfast and lunch the following day, have dinner, repeat. This is an every-other-day twenty-four hour fast. They are only skipping two meals every other day. Others prefer to eat 3 meals on day one and nothing at all on day two, then back to three meals on day three. This is a thirty-six hour fast. Fasting has no set schedule, only you determine when to eat and when to fast.

Various methods

Some choose to do a 24 hour fast (going from lunch to lunch, dinner to dinner, etc.) a few times per week. This is beneficial, however, it's a slower process. Doing this on a daily basis has shown remarkable gains both in terms of weight loss and insulin reduction.

Some choose to fast for 48 hours one time per week, every week. This means, for example, you would eat your last meal at dinner on Monday, don't eat Tuesday, skip breakfast and lunch on Wednesday then eat dinner Wednesday evening.

Some choose to fast for 3-7 days per month.

Some choose to fast for 2 weeks a year or even a few times in a year.

For the purpose of weight loss and insulin reduction, fasting will have a quicker response and be more effective if done daily or by doing a seven to fourteen day extended fast. Not everyone wants to jump right into it, however, I have noticed that those who try to do it more slowly, by starting with an eight-hour eating window then gradually shortening feels it's like starting over each step of the way. Remember you are establishing when you will be hungry, if you keep changing it you will be hungry when you don't want to be. Go for the gusto and do one meal per day for a fast change in health and weight status.

On the following page you will find some example schedules of eating for various fasting regimens. Remember, these are just examples and you will need to find what times and methods work best for you and your lifestyle. Flexibility is key, you can change things up as you go, just remember that your body will need some time to catch up and know when to be hungry.

The hours of fasting are counted as the hours between the last meal of one day and the next meal, regardless of whether you eat again the next morning or 3 days later. If you are finding it hard to fit a regular fasting schedule into your daily life due to lifestyle, work, or any other reason, use the flexibility of fasting and create a schedule that works for you. A personalized schedule may be 20 hours fasting Monday and Thursday, 18 on Saturday and Sunday, and 24 on Tuesday and Wednesday. It's okay to switch things up throughout the week or as you need to. Life happens, roll with it.

Example 1 – every other day 24 hour fast

MON	TUES	WED	THUR	FRI	SAT	SUN
Lunch		Lunch		Lunch		Lunch
Dinner	Dinner	Dinner	Dinner	Dinner	Dinner	Dinner

Example 2 – 36 hour fast

MON	TUES	WED	THUR	FRI	SAT	SUN
Lunch		Lunch		Lunch		Lunch
Dinner		Dinner		Dinner		Dinner

Example 3 – 42 hour fast

MON	TUES	WED	THUR	FRI	SAT	SUN
Lunch		Lunch		Lunch		
Dinner		Dinner		Dinner	Dinner	

Example 4 – 48 hour fast

MON	TUES	WED	THUR	FRI	SAT	SUN
Lunch						
Dinner		Dinner		Dinner		Dinner

Many people will find it easier to begin fasting if they are already eating a ketogenic diet (high fat, moderate protein, low carbohydrate) as they are already "fat adapted" and their body is used to burning fat for fuel. I have heard others not on any particular type of diet say it made no difference for them at all; fasting was either easy or a little hard in the beginning, but never impossible. It is true that if you consume higher fat and protein content than carbohydrates during your earing window you will be satiated longer. Having a Bullet Proof coffee (with grass-fed butter and MCT oil) during your eating window can definitely keep you full for hours.

Eating healthy, whole foods, during your feasting time is best, but it's true you can lose weight fasting while eating nothing but junk. This is not advised though, for obvious reasons. I personally tested this theory that you could eat whatever you wanted to and still lose weight. I ate, daily, fast food and junk food for six months. Occasionally I would have a "decent" meal in a restaurant (who really knows if it was "decent") on the weekend with a frozen margarita and an hour or so later have popcorn and M&Ms at the movie. During the work week, I ate fast food, gas station pizza, restaurant foods, etc. Sometimes I even ate a pint of Ben & Jerry's for lunch All high carb, high sugar, high octane... and plenty of additives.

Did I lose weight during all this madness? You bet I did. Twenty-one pounds in roughly six months. That's not a lot for 6 months, when others doing the same amount of fasting may have lost forty, fifty and over 75 pounds in that amount of time, but when you consider what I ate it was remarkable. It was the easiest weight loss I have ever experienced. I did not deny myself anything and I wasn't hungry outside of my eating window. After about 4-5 months I began to crave vegetables and meat, my body was telling me what it needed. But it *worked.* Why did it work if I was eating all the garbage food? Because I had approximately 20-24 hours per day of clean fasting. I would be remiss if I failed to mention that my lab results after 6 months were frightening. My inflammation level increased, as did just about all my lipids (that alone can be explained by the process of fat breakdown releasing into the blood stream). The high inflammation is what I found most disturbing. I knew that even though I was losing fat I was gaining risk due to a poor diet. How did I lose weight eating high caloric, high refined carbohydrate, high sugar junk food every day?

Clean fasting is where the magic happens. During the fasting time as your insulin decreases your growth hormone increases and your body begins a process called autophagy. In 2016 the Nobel Prize in Physiology or Medicine was awarded to Yoshinori Ohsumi for his work on autophagy. From the Greek words *auto* meaning "self" and *phagein* to eat, you can see that autophagy quite literally means to eat oneself.

With Ohsumi's work comes a new and better understanding of autophagy and the important physiological functions it commands. Cells have a variety of components such as organelles and proteins that can be damaged or dysfunctional and autophagy provides for those components to be destroyed and recycled. It provides a rapid response to fuel needs for energy and the renewal of the discarded and damaged cellular components. Following an infection, autophagy helps to eliminate and remove the offending viruses and bacteria. When the cells use autophagy to rid the body of the damaged proteins it counteracts the damage of aging.

When people do intermittent daily fasting and autophagy kicks in you can see a huge difference in their appearance verses someone who simply loses a lot of weight. When someone loses a lot of weight, they typically have saggy skin, appear older and maybe even unwell. Weight loss with fasting and supercharged autophagy produces the opposite effect. People appear younger, healthier, more radiant and without sagging skin. Remarkably, even lose neck skin can tighten up with autophagy. It helps organs become healthier and function improves and there is even an element of anti-aging associated. This is seen not only in the skin but also at the cellular level.

Of interest, a study done by Marinac, et al. states, "The cohort of 2413 women (mean [SD] age, 52.4 [8.9] years) reported a mean (SD) fasting duration of 12.5 (1.7) hours per night. In repeated-measures Cox proportional hazards regression models, fasting less than 13 hours per night (lower 2 tertiles of nightly fasting distribution) was associated with an increase in the risk of breast cancer recurrence compared with fasting 13 or more hours per night". Fast longer for greater risk reduction?

One of the remarkable things with fasting is the body re-composition that takes place. The scale may only see a few pounds difference but the patient may have dropped a few sizes in clothes. This is due to the re-composition of the tissue. Bones become denser and heavier, muscles become denser and heavier, and weight shifts. It can be seen even with simple daily fasting and no workouts. Obviously, including exercise is the healthier thing to do, but for the patient who is immobile or for other reasons can't exercise they can still get the benefits of autophagy. When the patient sees the changes in their body it is motivating and they feel rewarded for their effort. Remind them they may have slow times and they will need to remain patient and not expect changes to be constant just as their weight gain wasn't.

HOW TO CLEAN FAST

Clean fasting seems to create a lot of unnecessary confusion when people first begin. It's very clear and concise, not need to make it difficult. During the clean fasting time you can drink as much as you like but it must be limited to black coffee, black tea, green tea, still water or sparkling water with no added flavors. None. That's it, it's not hard but time and time again I get asked, "What about just a little cream in my coffee?" "What about the sparkling water with lime?" "What about......... it says no calories....?"

Calories don't matter, what matters is that anything you add, milk, cream, even artificial sweeteners, will spike your insulin. Insulin up isn't good; congratulations, you just ended your fast. If you don't like black coffee but feel you need the caffeine, try a pinch of pink salt to cut the bitterness. Purchase high quality beans and grind them yourself, then use the pour over technique. This often creates a milder, less bitter taste.

Your coffee taste preferences will change if you continue to drink the same thing daily; over time you may not like the old way if you try it. If you don't think you can drink black coffee, switch to green or black tea. Not herbal tea, that isn't really tea. Just green or black tea. Hot, cold, it doesn't matter. Many people who don't enjoy the taste of black coffee do enjoy it cold. Same with tea. Sparkling water is a good way to get over a soda addiction and make you feel a bit full. You still get the fizz without the insulin spike. Be careful though, the carbonation can make some people have an increased appetite. If you find you are hungry after drinking sparkling water stop drinking it until your insulin level has decreased, this can be days, weeks, or months depending on how quickly your insulin level drops.

Coffee and green tea both have a small appetite decreasing effect that may help with hunger in the first few days. Over time your body will become used to not eating during your fasting time and you may not feel you need (or want) to continue drinking it. Many people choose to continue for the other health properties contained within the beverages as well as a comfortable ritual.

FASTING FOR DIABETICS

If you have type 2 diabetes you can still fast, however, you should always consult with your medical provider before making any dietary changes. If your health care provider is not familiar (or supportive) of intermittent fasting for diabetics please search for one who is.

I like to use seven to fourteen day fasts for severe diabetics and a thirty-six hour fast three times per week in the beginning for pre-diabetic, mild or moderate diabetics. This schedule stays the same until the insulin levels have dropped, blood sugars have stabilized, the patient is off all medication, their weight is where desired and they are no longer considered diabetic. Medications are stopped (or reduced) during the extended fast with blood sugar being monitored frequently. Once these things are achieved the patient will switch (if desired) to a fasting schedule that fits with their lifestyle and they are able to maintain the changes. This schedule of fasting three times per week may only be needed for a few weeks to a few months; it's dependent on the patient's response. Often the longer a patient has been diagnosed with diabetes the longer it takes; but not always. Some reversals can happen quickly even when diabetic for over twenty years and on insulin.

What is eaten during this reversal process is far more crucial for those with diabetes than those without. It's imperative that you remove sugar and other refined carbohydrates from your diet. This alone will jump start your reversal and make it easier for you to fast. There are many books and internet sites created specifically for those on a ketogenic diet and you will find a massive amount of information for food choices, recipes and support.

The thirty-six hour fast is simply not eating for one day. This means you eat your meals as usual (high fat, moderate protein and low carbohydrate) with dinner on Monday being your last meal of the day. Tuesday you don't eat. Wednesday you eat again as normal. Thursday you don't eat, Friday you eat etc. Be mindful of what and when you put in your mouth on the days you eat as this will affect the rate of reversal. Sticking to the ketogenic diet is easy if you are prepared and have meals ready or ready to cook on your feasting days. Snacking isn't necessary and this unhealthy habit needs to stop; the sooner you stop snacking the better!

On fasting days, you need to reduce or stop any medication that is designed to lower your blood sugar level. Your blood sugar will naturally decrease due to no food intake during this time. It is recommended to check your blood sugar levels three to four times daily. Please be sure to do this under the direction of your medical provider. I have seen patients go off all diabetes related medications within a few weeks when they use the fasting and feasting protocols.

EXTENDED FASTING

Extended fasts are those fasts which are over forty-eight hours to an indefinite number of days. I don't recommend going over fourteen days for a variety of reasons but if you choose to do so please only do this with your medical providers supervision. Extended fasts can help when you hit a plateau, have gone off your fasting schedule, or just want to boost your autophagy and ketones. Regarding ketones; exogenous, supplemental ketones can be beneficial to brain health and improve leptin (the satiety hormone) sensitivity.

During the extended fasts I recommend that you ingest more than water as you need electrolytes and sodium. Drinking bone broth twice daily is a good and healthy way to keep in balance. I do not recommend drinking distilled or "Smart" water during an extended fast as the lack of sodium in distilled water can cause dehydration as it pulls sodium out of the cells for balance.

After an extended fast it's best to restart eating slowing. Start with something small and light, gradually go back to your normal daily or

every other day, fasting schedule. Resist the urge to overeat! Breaking your fast with a glass of water before you eat can be helpful to overcome the urge to consume too much. Overeating after an extended fast won't hurt you but can be very uncomfortable and you may need to spend quite a lot of time in the bathroom.

EXERCISE WHILE FASTING

There is no reason to stop or change your exercise routine because of fasting. As long as you have fat stores on your body you will not be deprived of energy. Many athletes work out in the fasted state because of the benefits derived from low insulin. Increased adrenaline during the fasting time stimulates the body to begin breaking down fat and utilizing it for energy. When actor Hugh Jackman needed to gain muscle for his role in the Marvel Comic film, Wolverine, he turned to intermittent fasting. Remember that growth hormone is increased during the fasted state and this helps with muscle growth and development.

FEASTING

What should I eat? Can I eat what I want? How much should I eat? Should I count calories? As I mentioned previously, eating what you want can lead to weight loss but certainly isn't the healthiest thing to do if what you want consists of highly refined and processed foods. Considering that you are working at lowering insulin, you need to think about what I am about to tell you then adjust your food as you feel appropriate.

Refined carbohydrates raise your insulin level the fastest and the highest. The higher the level the longer it takes to come down and go into fat burning. Eliminating sugar and as many refined carbohydrates (breads, pasta, cereal, etc.) from your diet will be very beneficial, but if you have type 2 diabetes it's crucial. Those with diabetes need to eat a diet rich in healthy fat, moderate protein and low in carbohydrates. Removing the refined carbohydrates and eliminating sugar is a must in the beginning for diabetics.

Proteins are next in terms of insulin spike. It's not quite as high as carbohydrates but it's a moderate spike. With both protein and carbohydrates, the more you eat the higher the insulin spike. Animal proteins are fine, we now know that the saturated fat in them is not going to cause cardiovascular disease. Saturated fats can increase the large, fluffy (healthy) LDL and HDL, but does not increase the small, dense (bad) LDL. Refined carbohydrate will increase the small, dense, (bad) LDL. Keep in mind that excess protein is processed by the liver and stored as fat so you don't want to exceed more than about 30% of your diet in protein.

Dietary fat is interesting in that it seems to have a cap, a limit on the how high it will spike insulin. The more you eat does not affect the level of insulin, it remains the same. Eating healthy high fat is satiating, good for your weight loss and overall health. Avocados once demonized for being so high in fat are now known to be extremely healthy. Eating fat, both saturated and monounsaturated is associated with a lower risk of total mortality. Higher saturated fat diets are associated with lower risk of stroke, and total fat, whether saturated or unsaturated, is not associated with heart attack or death from cardiovascular disease. And to top it off, refined carbohydrate intake *is* associated with a higher total mortality risk. Looking at all the low-

fat diet hype to reduce heart attacks now seems almost a crime!

*A list of healthy food choices can be found in a later chapter.

Open your eating window with whatever you choose; many prefer to open with a high fat option because the insulin spike is lower and they feel fuller which in turns means they eat less. Not everyone does this and you don't have to either, but it is an option. You may open your window with the same thing each day or switch it up; there is no hard-fast rule here. Your eating window can also be longer or shorter from day to day, but don't make it too long or you will lose the benefit of autophagy and the fasting time.

I can't stress enough how eating "whatever you want" isn't always what's the healthiest thing to do and could be detrimental. There are fasting groups on the internet that promote the "eat what you want" mantra and still lose weight and they aren't wrong. They are, however, ill-advised as fasting is not a cure all, it won't provide you with the proper nutrients needed to maintain health. Eating whatever you want is absolutely a good thing if what you want are nutritious, whole foods. Everybody is different and while eating non-nutritious foods may be okay for some, it's not for all.

Should you be permitted to eat dessert and celebrate with elaborate feasting? Absolutely! We will always feast big, just don't do it all the time. Make it special. We associate time with friends and family with food, holidays with food, funerals with food, birthdays, anniversaries, and promotions with food. Even when sick your mom wants to bring you food. You need to establish routines that do not always include food with loved ones. Save the big feasting for special times, not Saturday brunch. Weekends are not holidays or days for celebration, stop that kind of thinking!

Eating until you feel satisfied will become easier the longer you do intermittent fasting. You will naturally begin to use "appetite correction" but you need to pay attention to your body. When we eat and feel full but continue to eat more, we are destroying our body's ability to recognize and tell the brain when we have had enough. When you override and ignore the signals long enough your body gets very confused and stops sending the signal that you are full. To achieve appetite correction, you need to stop eating when you feel satisfied. You may find that early on when your window opens you get full faster, sometimes this happens and sometimes it doesn't. You don't have to eat the same amount each day; if you aren't satisfied eat, if you are, stop eating. Allow your body the time and opportunity to relearn hunger and satiety signals.

CALORIES

Counting calories is useless. Your body has receptors for proteins and fat, but, not surprisingly, there isn't a single calorie receptor to be found in the body. Dr. Jason Fung, a Toronto Nephrologist, made the obviously facetious comparison when he asked if eating 1000 calories of broccoli would have the same effect as eating 1000 calories of sugar. Of course not! The sugar, as you know, will be converted to fat and increase inflammation but not the broccoli. Calories are not all the same and your body is smart enough to know this. How food is processed in your body defies the old, useless theory of "calories in vs calories out" for weight loss. Basically, calories are not part of physiology.

I saw, again, someone posting online about needing a calorie deficit to lose weight, saying it's the law of thermodynamics (the second law of thermodynamics states that the total entropy of an isolated system can never decrease over time) and you can't dispute it. Well, you can dispute it because the human body is not an isolated or closed system!

Energy is used in so many different ways within the body and, again, your body is smart and is not going to allow you to use more energy than you take in for long. After a while of consuming less than you burn, your body will begin conserving energy so that your output is the same as your input. It will slow your metabolic processes, decrease your core body temperature, slow your heart rate, etc. Essentially you will lower your metabolism but your weight, even with lower calories, will begin its climb back up to your weight set point. Once you hit the previous weight set point it continues to rise because your metabolism is slower than it was at that weight before you trashed your metabolism. Eating for a "caloric deficit" is okay for a very short-term goal, but anything beyond that will leave a body cold, tired, and fatter. Wait, what is a weight set point?

The weight set point is where your hormones sustain a targeted weight. So, say you weight right around 187 pounds for 5 years, your weight set point is 187 pounds. Now, say you go on a low-calorie diet, a low-fat diet, or other restrictive diet, with or without exercise. The weight goes down but the insulin remains up, keeping your weight set point in place. Your body's hormones will drive your weight back up to that set point. When you have created a situation to slow your basal metabolism, your weight will increase over the previous set point because you now require fewer calories to maintain the weight you once were for so long.

A good example of this is the show Fit to Fat to Fit where trainers go from a healthy weight, gain to an unhealthy weight and lose it again. They like to show how easy it is; but this is false. They gained the weight in a very short amount of time; their weight set point probably didn't move much if at all. It's far easier to lose the weight that you have had for a short time than it is to lose it after being overweight or obese for years.

Another example: If you were used to spending $100 per day, every day, and suddenly your income dropped by a third you may not mind immediately and keep the same spending habits. But soon you would notice your account balance going down and you would decrease your spending so you didn't have to sell your belongings to survive. Your body is really smart when it comes to budgeting and rationing. When it realizes you aren't taking in as much it will stop putting out as much in order to conserve.

Calories are managed differently depending on what they are comprised of. Protein and Carbohydrates are taken to the liver for processing, fat does not go through the liver. Excess carbohydrates equal high insulin which locks down fat burning and creates fat stores and triglycerides. Yet you can eat excess fat, consuming far more calories, without causing a high insulin spike and the body switches to fat burning. This is exactly what you want! Leave the old myth of calories in calories out where it belongs, in the past.

SNACKING

Snacking is unnecessary and dangerous to your health. Why do you snack? Why do you think you need to snack? Do you really believe your body needs to have something every couple of hours in order to survive? Children don't even need snacks. A newborn baby is perfectly content going 3-4 hours between meals (less if breast fed) without a "snack" between bottles. If a seven-pound human can go four hours, can you not go 6 or 8 or 12? Yes, you can.

Snacking after breakfast, after lunch, after dinner and even bedtime is routine for many children and adults. As you have already learned, this constant fueling of the body leads to a sustained, high insulin level. You didn't get this way over night; it takes years of eating this way before suddenly the weight starts piling on and you are unable to lose it like you once could.

So called "healthy snacks" often consists of foods laden with high fructose corn syrup, table sugar, and refined carbohydrates These foods need to eliminate from your diet except for during times of celebration and always preceded or followed by (or both) clean fasting.

If you are diabetic and say you need to snack to keep your blood sugar from dropping doesn't it make more sense to not snack and lower your glucose level naturally? Yes, it does. You don't have a disease of low blood sugar, it's a disease of high insulin. Remember to consult with your medical provider before you make adjustments to your medication.

WHAT ABOUT CHILDREN?

Children should not be put on a fasting plan. Have you noticed that young children will regulate the amount they eat by often refusing a meal because they aren't hungry? When that happens what do parents tend to do? They argue, convince and even threaten the child into eating. Society seems to have this idea that you absolutely just can't skip a meal! If the child isn't hungry don't force them; remember the principles of appetite correction? If you force the body to eat when it's not hungry you are going to mess up the hormone production that regulates both hunger and satiety. If they aren't eating and are losing weight seek the advice of your medical provider as there may be an underlying reason.

What you should do is feed them whole, healthy foods low in natural sugar and remove all foods with added sugars. It's also imperative to remove snacking. All snacking. Snacks are usually not very nutritious, contain sweeteners that lead to disease, and keep the child's insulin levels high. Their body is no different in that regard, you must prevent them from creating a sustained, high insulin environment in order to prevent obesity and diabetes. It's the same for children in terms of appetite creation; the more often you eat the more often you are hungry.

Also remove all soda and fruit juices. Some of these juices, especially from concentrate with no sugar added are still 60% fructose! Adding water to equal 50% of the volume in regular juice (not made from concentrate) is a good way to decrease sugars while curbing the taste for so much sweetness. There is no reason to get children addicted to the sugary flavors that will only lead to a negative outcome.

Raise your children with plenty of vegetables, berries, meats, healthy fats and a lot of pure, clean water. Make meal time a social time around the table. Make it a habit to only eat at the table but not make food the center of attraction; make being together talking to one another the main thing. Wait, isn't that what they used to do way back when? Oh yeah, before weight gain and obesity. Before there was a fast food joint on every corner. Before gummy fruit snacks. Before juice boxes. Before Coke became the drink of choice. Before eating became the primary activity.

WHOOSH!

You may have heard the term "whoosh" in regard to weight loss, it actually can and does happen. When fat cells empty their contents, it is quickly replaced with water. This water acts like a place holder in anticipation of the fat contents returning. After a time of no fat returning the cells release the fluid and the body has a "whoosh" of fluid lost and the scale goes down.

TIPS AND TRICKS

There are some things that you can do to enhance weight loss and insulin reduction. One of those things is to use apple cider vinegar. Apple cider vinegar contains acetic acid which has many health benefits including lowering inflammation, appetite suppression, increasing metabolism, may help eliminate heartburn, helps with bad breath, reduces water retention, lowers blood pressure, and causes decreases in both blood glucose and insulin spikes.

Two teaspoons (in water) or two capsules of apple cider vinegar has been shown to decrease hunger. When consumed just prior to a meal containing refined carbohydrates and again just after the meal, glucose and insulin spikes can be reduced by approximately 34%. Adding fiber capsules before a meal can decrease the insulin spike even further.

Type 2 diabetics can benefit by consuming in either liquid or capsule form of the apple cider vinegar at night before bed which seems to cause a decline in high morning blood sugar.

Consuming peanut products can reduce glycemic response by about 55%. Eating more foods that cause less of an insulin spike can assist in getting that sustained high insulin lowered.

Take a look at a sample of the insulin index.

The Insulin Index

Butter	2	Turkey	23
Coconut Oil	3	Chicken	23
Flax Oil	3	Whole Milk	40
Pecans	5	Beef	51
Avocado	6	Scallops	59
Cream Cheese (not low-fat)	8	Crisps (chips)	61
Bacon	9	Brown Rice	62
Pork	11	Apple	75

Peanut Butter	11	Low Fat Yogurt	76
Cod	12	Fat Free Pretzel	81
Duck	12	Banana	84
Peanuts	13	Crackers	86
Pork Sausage	13	Whole-wheat Bread	90
Cheddar Cheese	15	White Bread	100
Chia Seeds	15	Baked Beans	100
Egg Yolk	16	Sweetened Yogurt	115
Coleslaw	20	Potatoes	121
Whole Egg	21	Jelly Beans	160

As you can see by the insulin index chart, eating a banana or apple is going to raise your insulin level markedly higher than cream cheese, bacon, peanut butter, or even chips. Milk, while low on the glycemic index is actually much higher on the insulin index. The ADA recommends utilizing the glycemic index to choose foods that don't raises glucose levels too much; remember, we aren't treating hyperglycemia, we are treating hyperinsulinemia!

Adding vinegar to rice during or after preparation then refrigerating it until cold considerably reduces the glycemic load and subsequent insulin spike. This effect is not lost upon reheating. This holds true for potatoes as well. Cooking them, refrigerating them, and eating cold as in a potato salad with a bit of vinegar or reheating them both have a lower glycemic/insulin reaction.

FIBER

During the days when food began to change another thing happened that boosted the obesity epidemic; wheat processing. Wheat was once eaten in a semi whole state including the hull, bran and germ. The germ is full of nutritious fatty acids while the hull and bran contain nutrients and fiber. After removal of those important components, the remaining wheat body is ground down and processed into a fine powder. The powder, which we know of as flour, is readily absorbed into the blood stream and spikes insulin instantly. Think about the cocaine user, they don't want a chunky product to snuff into their nose, they want a fine powder that can be absorbed quickly.

We have stretch receptors in our stomach which send signals to the

brain indicating fullness when eating. Without fiber, however, the stomach doesn't expand enough for these stretch receptors to signal the brain until the stomach contents are at a level that the bulk of food is determining fullness. We have hormones that tell our brain when we have had enough fat and hormones to tell our brain when we have had enough protein, but we are lacking in one that recognizes our refined carbohydrate intake. This is why you can be too full for more meat but still have room for cake.

Think about this; without fiber to expand the stomach you can pack a lot of refined carbohydrate in there and it's not going to expand until you are literally full. Consider a balloon that you fill with a half cup of fiber then add water. The balloon will expand far more than that half cup of content. Now take another balloon and pour flour into it. It's not going to expand until you have a lot of flour in there. Add water and it doesn't cause the same expansion. So basically, you can eat a lot more refined carbohydrate than you can natural, fiber containing foods.

Fiber is one of the things that can help decrease obesity; it is protective

in that way. Fiber is the difference between carbohydrates in vegetables and carbohydrates in ice cream or other refined foods with a high carbohydrate count. It has been said that if carbohydrate were a poison, fiber is the antidote. All foods in nature that contain carbohydrates likewise contain fiber. It's when this fiber is removed from our diets that trouble begins. What can you do?

Adding fiber into your diet is the answer. It won't reduce your colon cancer risk as once hypothesized, but it will reduce your insulin spike. So, if type 2 diabetes is a result of sustained high insulin, and fiber can lower insulin levels, wouldn't the addition of more fiber in the diet be beneficial to diabetics? Absolutely, and there are multiple studies to back this fact up.

A diet with a high glycemic response but low in fiber can increase the risk of type 2 diabetes by as much as 76%! A later study in men showed an increase in risk of 217%! This type of diet is reproduced in the very foods consumed most often; those with a lot of refined carbohydrate and sugar with little fiber content. The addition of cereal fiber (found in whole grains, brown rice, seeds, barley, etc. were shown to be more

protective than fiber from fruits and vegetables.

Taking a fiber capsule prior to meals containing refined carbohydrates will help counteract the insulin spike and help with satiety by activating stretch receptors at the same time. Of course, it's best to not eat the refined carbohydrates and eat only whole grains instead, but until that time get some fiber capsules and work on reducing your refined carbohydrate intake.

A FEW WORDS ABOUT GLUTEN

You've likely heard people complaining about the "gluten free craze" and maybe had that internal eye rolling at people who do not have celiac disease but are on a gluten free diet. Glutens are the sticky substance that gives bread it's strength and elasticity, without gluten it's heavy and dense. Gluten, however, is very inflammatory (and leads to insulin resistance) and most people have sensitivities to it but don't know it. We typically think of intestinal issues related to gluten, but that's not always the case. Migraines, multiple sclerosis (MS) misdiagnosis, amyotrophic lateral sclerosis (ALS or Lou Gehrig's disease) misdiagnosis, tremors, fibromyalgia, etc., have been associated with gluten sensitivity. Gluten sensitivity can affect pancreatic cells which affects insulin production and function. It would do the majority of us good to eat gluten free foods.

BMI & BATHROOM SCALES

Anytime I am in a lecture at a medical conference and they start basing their information on BMI I tune them out. BMI stands for Body Mass Index and is being used as a tool to measure fatness and therefore disease risk. I urge you to not rely on BMI, there is really no reason to use it at all when trying to reduce weight. Why? Because BMI=BS.

Obesity is no longer just a social issue, it's a health crisis. Medical science, through many painstaking years of research, has taught us that obesity is related to more chronic and often fatal health maladies than previously recognized. From heart disease, diabetes, cancer, osteoarthritis, gout, sleep apnea, to asthma and more, the cost to American's physically, emotionally and financially is staggering. With obesity at epidemic proportions in the United States it makes sense for medical providers to address this health problem with their patients, but are we doing more harm than good? Is our methodology, using this BMI chart, based on good science or are we relying on something that is physiologically baseless?

Body Mass Index (BMI), simply put, does not accurately reflect a level of fatness or obesity. BMI is a 200-year-old formula being used in the United States who, ironically, prides themselves on their technology and progressive medical science as world leading.

Many practitioners have been taught by medical educators and in turn repeat to their patients that BMI is an accurate measure of fatness; this declaration is grossly misleading and false. The CDC states the BMI is only "moderately" correlated with more direct measures of body fat, yet continues to make health recommendations and base obesity rates on this outdated formula.

Starting with the calculation in dissection of the formula you should ask yourself, why is a person's height squared for this calculation? This makes no sense. Unless the outcome doesn't fit the theory, therefore you must change the formula until it does. Similar to what many people believe Ancel Keys did in his infamous 7 Country Study in 1958; eliminate the countries from the study if they may disprove the hypothesis.

The founder of the BMI calculation, Lambert Quatelet, stated this formula should never be used to measure a level of body fat as it is not appropriate for that use as it does not give an accurate measure of fatness. He was a mathematician not a physician, but he knew that bone weighs more than muscle which weighs twice as much as fat; factors that render this formula inaccurate for measuring fatness.

The BMI does not take into consideration the age, gender, or muscle mass of the patient. Bone density will vary from person to person and a low BMI could indicate that the bones are not dense, even diseased, but because the BMI falls in the normal range this can lead the practitioner to assume the patient is healthier than they may be. An average or low BMI could be indicative of very low muscle mass; it doesn't always mean the patient is at a healthy level of fatness. Just as bone density is not the same for all patients, muscle mass varies from person to person and a BMI does not differentiate between a pound/kilogram of muscle vs fat vs bone. For example, men who are in the United States Army Special Forces unit have BMI that categorizes them as obese when in fact they have very little body fat, whereas another person of the same height and weight might actually be clinically obese.

After years of teaching female patients about breast health, cancer, and preventative measures, breast self-exams for average risk women have been discouraged. Studies reflected women had increased stress levels and feelings of guilt for not doing them. The consensus was that advising women to conduct a monthly exam was of little value and potentially harmful. The risks were determined to outweigh the benefits as it was determined that breast cancer morbidity was falsely elevated resulting in more unnecessary mammograms and biopsies. These procedures aren't without potential risks to the health of the woman, not to mention the associated costs. The bottom line was that putting women at risk of harm without any decrease in breast cancer death rates didn't equate to an evidenced based rationale. Eliminating breast self-exams is an excellent example of how we need to weigh the risks against the benefits and decide if what we are doing is a productive and positive methodology. That needs to be measured against creating an environment of potential harm. So, what does this have to do with BMI?

BMI numbers can create stress in people when discovering their "score" whether via health care practitioner or on online BMI calculator. This is not unlike the stress measured in the breast self-exam study. Further, the woman with dense, healthy bones, average or low body fat and healthy muscle mass may sacrifice nutrition by restricting calories unnecessarily. Does she need to lose weight? Perhaps not, but she was just informed she is over-weight or obese based on BMI.

Clinicians who counsel patients for weight loss based on these arbitrary BMI numbers are likely not practicing responsibly. They are not treating the patient, they are treating a number that is affected by, but not accommodating to, individual body composition. Counseling clinically overweight and obese patients on the dangers of refined carbohydrates, sedentary lifestyles, lack of healthy dietary fats, lack of restorative sleep, and increased stress may be a more effective strategy. Familiarizing oneself with current nutritional research the clinician can help the patient develop pathways to realistic goals.

Bathroom scales and weighing daily is another no-no. The human body is not one big blob of fat, so when you step on a scale you are not weighing fat content, you are weighing fat, skin, muscle, bone, cartilage, organs, intracellular fluids, extracellular fluids (approximately

15 liters), lymphatic fluids, blood volume, urine, cerebral spinal fluid, and poop! Now if you step on the scale today and weight 183 pounds and tomorrow you weight 182, did you lose a pound of fat? Maybe, but do you really know? No, you don't. The next day you weight 185 pounds, did you gain two pounds of fat? Maybe but do you really know? Nope. Maybe you are retaining fluid, maybe your bones and muscles are getting denser, maybe you have more poop...

The reality of it is you don't know what exactly you are weighing and it's likely going to play games with your head. This is why people who fast daily can see their body changing shape and dropping sizes in clothing without seeing the scale budge much.

When changes are or are not seen on a day to day basis, or that aren't steadily decreasing, the consequences can impact the resolve to continue on the reversal program. You may feel down, feel like it's failing, that it doesn't work for you and even give up on the program all together. The best thing you can do is throw out the scales or put them away and weigh next year. Don't base your weight reversal on unclear, fluid measurements. If you feel you must keep a record of the loss use a measuring tape and measure upper arms, chest, high waist, low waist, buttocks, thighs, and calves. You may see inches lost long before you see pounds gone on a bathroom scale. It took your body some time to raise your insulin levels to the point you gained fat or became insulin resistant, you have to allow your body time to reverse that process. Remember, you can jumpstart the process of reversal with the ketogenic diet and extended fasts of three to 14 days.

If you aren't seeing changes over time you may need to have some other lab tests ordered to see if your thyroid and other hormones are functioning at optimal levels. Suboptimal levels can result in failure to lose weight. See Part 2 on hormones.

BEGIN!

To begin healing your body you must prepare your mind as well. You need to do whatever it takes to let go of old thoughts, old information, old habits and be at peace with your decision to make this change. Take a week or so to prepare by planning your fast times and your meals, or jump right in to a three or more day fast. During that fasting time make your plan, set your goals. The choice is yours on how you want to proceed.

Schedule an appointment to have labs done if you need to; not everyone does but it's helpful to have an idea of where you are nutritionally and hormonally. Sometimes the lab results themselves are motivating either to get started or keep going when you see great things happening.

Decide how you want to measure your accomplishments; there are many, many ways. The scale, as discussed, isn't always the best way to measure weight loss. It can be very misleading and may thwart your progress if you feel you aren't getting anywhere. There are many non-scale victories to count! Clothes fit better or become too big, appetite correction kicked in, you are craving healthier foods, lab results are looking better, skin is looking less old and tired, people may compliment your appearance more. Your sleep and moods may have improved, your performance at work and your relationships with others may have improved. There are countless ways in which your body can tell you that healing is happening.

You will find, unfortunately, that others will condemn your plan by telling you it's unhealthy; it's going to make you burn muscle, it will put you into starvation mode, it will lower your metabolism, it will make you get ulcers... I tell my patients to not let it get to them and simply say, "I am working at lowering my insulin levels for health reasons, weight loss is just a beautiful side effect." If that doesn't work ask them if they want your fat clothes.

It's not always easy to educate others, they, like the rest of us, believed the diet gurus when they told us how horrible it would be for our bodies if we skipped a meal. Over time they will see that it's working for you, you look and feel great, and maybe, just maybe, they will make some of their own changes. You could always share a copy of this book, but do so carefully as to not offend.

WHAT IF I'M NOT LOSING WEIGHT?

You know the old saying, "You didn't gain it in a few days, you can't expect to lose it that way either"? It's true but there's even more. Remember, it took a long time of cellular level processing that caused weight gain long before you noticed it on your body or scale. The longer you have been overweight, the more insulin resistant or have higher sustained levels of insulin, and the more you have trashed your metabolism with low calorie dieting the longer it's going to take. Just because you aren't seeing rapid results doesn't mean your body isn't hard at work undoing the damage. When you gained weight, you didn't notice a change every single day, or every week, or even every month. Don't expect to see a decrease or change every day, every week, or even every month. Your body has to reverse that entire process that caused you to gain weight to start with.

With that being said; once you have spent time cleaning up your food choices, you have practiced appetite correction, you are active to help increase your metabolism, and you are sticking to a clean fast and still not losing – change it up.

Try alternate day fasting.

Try 2-3 days per week where you just don't eat at all.

Move your eating window, if it was in the evening try eating earlier in the day.

Shorten your window.

Drink more water.

Eat less protein and carbs.

Recheck your clean fast – are you actually sabotaging it and don't know it gum, mints, or something else?

Stop eating your favorite thing that you eat regularly for a week or two and see if your weight begins to move again.

Get more sleep.

Meditate to relieve stress – daily.

Fasting is one of the most effective ways to restore a body to health. In the animal world when sick they purposefully fast allowing the body to focus on healing rather than digestion. This is normal and natural.

Fasting is the quickest, healthiest, and most efficient way to reverse type 2 diabetes and obesity. Lowering insulin levels is the only way to do either successfully and sustainably; fasting does this and more.

Fasting is NOT starvation!

KETOGENIC DIET

The ketogenic diet is a high-fat, adequate (moderate) protein, low carbohydrate diet that in the medical arena has a long history. The ketogenic diet has been used effectively to treat difficult to control epilepsy in the pediatric population. It has also been used in cardiology to dramatically and quickly reduce cardiac risks. So why, you may ask, isn't it used more often in the event of obesity in the general patient population? I don't have an answer other than that of which was outlined earlier; the pushing of the low-fat, high carbohydrate, Standard American Diet.

When the "Atkins Diet" became popular there was a lot of controversy over its efficacy vs the efficacy of the low-fat diet. Of course, the low-fat diet paled in comparison to the weight loss and health gains seen with the Atkins Diet, but in the end neither have shown to be sustainable weight loss for various reasons; restrictive eating. That takes us back to the sustained loss with fasting and moving the insulin determined weight set point.

Lowering insulin and reversing insulin resistance is done fastest and most effectively through fasting. When incorporating the ketogenic diet, losses can be greater and health may improve for a variety of reasons; one being the lack of inflammation causing refined carbohydrates.

The ketogenic diet is a very low carbohydrate way of eating coupled with a moderate amount of high-quality proteins and healthy dietary fats. When carbohydrates are reduced the body enters a fat burning state which breaks down fats from both the food you eat and the fat stored in your body. During this process the body begins to produce ketone bodies and enters a state of ketosis. Do not confuse this with keto acidosis which is a completely different situation.

The benefits of a ketogenic diet are immense. Aside from fat loss there are other very beneficial changes. These changes can include:

- Improved mental clarity as the brain utilizes ketones for its primary fuel source instead of the glucose you eat. This can increase more nerve growth factors and synaptic connections which results in increased alertness, better focus, and improvement in cognitive function.
- Insulin metabolism in the body is improved with a low carbohydrate diet through the usage of the body breaking down fats and proteins.
- The utilization of body fat as fuel is why studies support this method for weight loss. Appetite and cravings are reduced for most people who stay on this way of eating.
- While the body is in ketosis it uses fat (both dietary and body) as fuel instead of the glucose derived from carbohydrate. Carbohydrates only give short bursts of energy where fat as fuel is sustained energy.
- Fatty acid metabolism is supported by the use of a ketogenic diet.

HOW TO EAT KETO

Discarding long standing eating habits isn't easy, nor is the idea of giving up certain foods permanently. This usually fails for obvious reasons. Use the ketogenic diet until your weight is where it should be then slowly add other foods while maintain an 8 hour or less eating window.

The recommended, but outdated, Standard American Diet looks much like this:

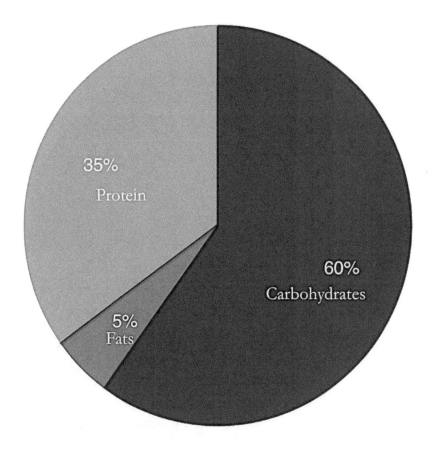

The typical vegetarian/vegan diet where consumers are simply using refined carbs in place of meat proteins:

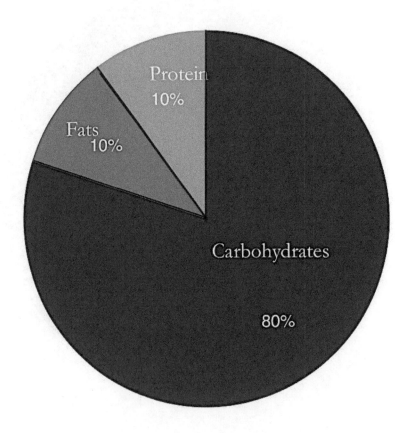

As you can see in the previous diagrams, the carbohydrate content is very high for both. Reducing the refined carbohydrate content will reduce inflammation and insulin resulting in better health and lower weight.

The ketogenic percentages look more like this (with variances):

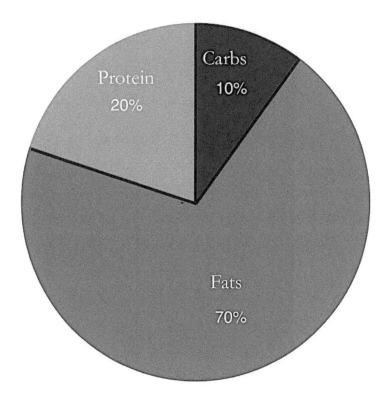

Adopting a ketogenic lifestyle can be overwhelming if you aren't prepared; just as any food restrictive diet is daunting when you are hungry and don't have readily available "allowed" foods. Prior to beginning a ketogenic lifestyle, you need to take time to learn about it, understand it, and then be prepared to embrace it. In general, we don't normally eat from a list of foods; we eat by meals made from recipes. If you try to eat a ketogenic diet by a food list you will most likely become bored quickly. The internet is full of websites, books, cookbooks, support groups, etc. where you can find a plethora of recipes and meal plans.

The keto diet doesn't work well for 100% of those who try it. Whether it's non-adherence or simply differences in food metabolism or sensitivities, or sustained high insulin levels, many people, especially women, claim it does not work for them. If it doesn't seem to be working for you the first thing you need to do is look at exactly what you are eating. You may be eating something that isn't actually keto friendly. If all seems okay perhaps you are eating something that your body is sensitive to, causing you to retain or shift fluids. For some, your insulin levels may be quite high and it will take longer to reverse them. I would suggest having a smaller eating window to combat this issue and get your body moving in the right direction.

The ketogenic diet restricts carbohydrates to 50 grams or below per day. If you think that is low, remember, there are essential fatty acids and essential proteins, but there are no essential carbohydrates!

The following is a list of foods by category to maintain this way of eating:

DAIRY

- Kefir, plain 1 cup
- Yogurt
  Plain full-fat/whole milk, Greek, ½ cup
- Milk, full-fat, 1 cup

PROTEIN

- Bacon, 2 slices
- Beef, all cuts, 3 oz
- Buffalo, 3 oz
- Cheese
  Feta, 2 oz
  Goat, 2 oz
  Mozzarella, 2 oz or ½ cup shredded
  Ricotta, 1/3 cup
  Cottage, ¾ cup
- Chicken, white or dark meat, 3 oz
- Cornish Hen, 4 oz
- Eggs, whole, 2
- Egg whites, 1 cp
- Elk, 3 oz
- Fish

Salmon, canned, fresh, or smoked 3 oz

Herring, 3 oz

Mackerel, 2 oz

Sardines, 3 oz

Trout, 4 oz

Tuna, canned, chunk light or solid light, water or oil, 4 oz

- Lamb, leg, chop or lean roast, 3 oz
- Liver, 3 oz
- Pork tenderloin, 3 oz
- Sausage, varies by type
- Shellfish, shrimp, crab, lobster, clams, mussels, oysters and scallops 4-5 oz

- Venison, 3 oz

VEGETABLES – NONSTARCHY

- Artichoke
- Asparagus
- Bamboo shoots
- Bean sprouts
- Bitter melon
- Bottle gourd
- Broccoli

- Brussel Sprouts
- Cabbage
- Cauliflower
- Celery
- Celery root
- Chayote
- Cucumber
  - Eggplant
  - Green or string beans
  - Hearts of palm
  - Jerusalem artichoke
  - Jicama
  - Kimchi
  - Kohlrabi
  - Leeks
  - Leafy greens (arugula, beets, collard, dandelion, endive, escarole, kale, spinach, Swiss chard, radicchio, watercress)
  - Lettuce (Boston, bibb, butter, frisee, grean leaf, red leaf, romaine)
  - Mushrooms
  - Okra

- Onions (green, brown, red, scallions, shallot, spring, white, yellow)
- Peppers (bell, jalapeño, poblano, sweet
- Radishes
- Rutabaga
- Sauerkraut
- Sea plants
- Sprouts
- Sugar snap peas, snow peas
- Summer squash (crookneck, delicata, yellow, spaghetti, zucchini, patty pan)
- Tomatoes
- Turnips
- Water chestnuts

For leafy greens a serving size is approximately 2-3 cups raw. For the rest: ½ cup cooked or 1 cup raw.

OILS AND FATS

- Avocado 2 Tbsp
- Avocado oil 1 tsp
- Butter 1 tsp
- Coconut milk
- Light, canned 3 Tbsp
- Regular, canned 1.5 Tbsp

- Coconut oil 1 tsp
- Cream 1 Tbsp
- Cream cheese 1 Tbsp
- Flaxseed oil 1 tsp
- Ghee/clarified butter 1 tsp
- Grapeseed oil 1 tsp
- Mayonnaise, unsweetened (avocado, grapeseed or olive oil 1 Tbsp
- MCT (medium chain triglyceride) oil 1 tsp
- MCT powder ½ Tbsp
- Olive oil, extra virgin 1 tsp
  - Olives, 8-10 medium or 6 large
  - Sesame oil 1 tsp
  - Sour cream 2 Tbsp

NUTS AND SEEDS

- Almonds 6
- Almond butter 1 ½ tsp
- Brazil 2
- Cashews 6
- Cashew butter 1 ½ tsp
- Chia seeds 1 Tbsp
- Coconut unsweetened, shredded 1 ½ Tbsp
- Flax seed, ground 1 ½ Tbsp

- Hazelnuts 5
- Hemp seeds 2 tsp
- Macadamia 3
- Pecans 4 halves
- Pine nuts 1 Tbsp
- Pistachios 12
- Pumpkin seeds 1 Tbsp
- Sesame seeds 1 Tbsp
- Sunflower seeds 1 Tbsp
- Tahini 1 ½ tsp
- Walnuts 4 halves

BEVERAGES (unlimited)

- Coffee/espresso unsweetened
- Green tea, unsweetened
- Non-caffeinated herbal teas (mint, chamomile, hibiscus, etc.)
- Mineral water (still or carbonated) except when fasting
- Sparkling water without artificial flavors
- Tap water, bottled water

CONDIMENTS, HERBS & SPICES (unlimited)

- Cacao powder/nibs
- Carob
- Black strap molasses
- Bone broth
- Flavored extracts (almond, vanilla)
- Garlic
- Ginger
- Herbs, all, fresh or dried
- Horseradish
- Hot sauce
- Lemon
- Lime
- Liquid amino acid
- Mustard
- Miso
- Salsa, unsweetened
- Soy sauce/tamari
- Spices, all, fresh or dried
- Tomato sauce, unsweetened
- Vinegar, unsweetened, organic apple cider, balsamic, red wine, white wine.

ALLOWED SWEETENERS

- Swerve
- Monk fruit extract

LEGUMES (occasional, they are a low-quality protein)

- Beans, (black eyed, black, cannellini, edamame, garbanzo, kidney, lima, mong, navy, pinto, etc.)
- Beans, vegetarian refried ½ cup
- Beans soups, homemade ¾ cup
- Hummus 4 Tbsp
- Lentils (brown, green, red, yellow, French) ½ cup, cooked
- Peas (pigeon, split) ½ cup, cooked
-

BERRIES

- Black Berries ¾ cup
- Blueberries ¾ cup
- Boysenberries ¾ cup
- Cranberries, unsweetened ½ cup
- Loganberries ¾ cup
- Raspberries 1 cup
- Strawberries 1 ¼ cup

AVOID

- Processed/sugary foods to include sauces such as soda, smoothies, ice cream, fruits juice, candies, etc.
- Fast food (pizza, burgers, chicken nuggets, pasta)
- Unhealthy fats such as processed vegetable oils
- Root vegetables and tubers such as potatoes, carrots
- Grains or starches and wheat based products like rice, pasta, cereal, bread, etc.
- Most fruit with the exception of a small amount of berries
- Low fat and diet products
- Alcoholic drinks that are sugary (some red wines are low in sugar and are keto friendly)
- Sugar free diet foods because they are often high in sugar alcohols or artificial sweeteners

HIDDEN CARBOHYDRATES

- Milk substitutes such as soy and almond milk often have hidden carbohydrates. Flavored milks usually contain more sugar.
- Chestnuts, most nuts and seeds have a little carbs but chestnuts contain around 6 to 7 g per serving.

- Yogurt, avoid low-fat and fruit flavored yogurt products. Use full fat or whole milk Greek yogurt instead.

- t or fat free often means the food contains more carbs due to added sugar for flavor.

- Ketchup and tomato sauces can contain hidden sugar and carbohydrates.

- Salad dressings, most contain sugar. Always check labels.

- No added sugar or sugar free foods that are naturally sweet like fruit juice or raisins are typically very high in sugar.

- Sugar comes with a variety of names, these include high fructose corn syrup, agave nectar, honey, molasses, and fridges concentrate.

MEAT BASED DIETS & KETOSIS

Carnivore diets, specifically those achieving a meat predominant or meat only based state of ketosis, are not healthy in the long term. While you may feel good due to the ketosis state, a meat-based ketosis is very inflammatory and meat protein in excess inhibits cellular repair. Remember too that excess protein is stored on the body as fat.

TIPS

Many people find a ketogenic diet to be constipating in the beginning. You can avoid this by adding fiber (powder, capsules, etc), magnesium supplements and by eating more leafy greens. MCT oil and avocado oil both have a natural laxative effect which can help. Drink plenty of water and move!

What is Keto flu? Symptoms that make up "keto flu" that happen in the early stages of restricting carbohydrates have a few different causes. Bone broth covers most!

Symptoms	What You Need	How to Get It
Dizziness	Sodium	Salt/Boullion
Headache	Sodium	"
Confusion	Sodium	"
Fatigue/Tiredness	Sodium	"
Restlessness	Sodium	"
Irritability	Sodium	"
Symptoms	**What You Need**	**How to Get It**
Irritability/anxiety	Magnesium	Magnesium supplement/TriSalts, seaweed/hemp seed
Lethargy	Magnesium	"
Confusion	Magnesium	"

Muscle Weakness	Magnesium	"
Muscle spasms and cramps	Magnesium	"
Impaired coordination	Magnesium	"
Vertigo	Magnesium	"
Difficulty swallowing	Magnesium	"

Symptoms	What you need	How to Get it
Dizziness	Potassium	Spinach, avocados, mushrooms, meat, TriSalts
Low blood pressure	Potassium	"
Nausea/vomiting	Potassium	"
Muscle weakness	Potassium	"
Fatigue	Potassium	"
Cramping	Potassium	"
Constipation/distention	Potassium	"

PART

TWO

HORMONES

MENOPAUSE

&

ANDROPAUSE

4

HORMONE BASICS

Just the mention of the word "hormone" elicits a response from some women (and medical providers) that I can only describe as horror. A number of these women are adamant that they do not want hormones rubbed on, injected into or implanted within their body. They want to age "naturally" and don't want the cancer that comes with estrogen replacement therapy. That would be perfectly understandable and reasonable if it were true, but it's not.

To understand where that myth came from you have to go back to the year 2002. A fifteen-year study into women's health was stopped three years early due to a preliminary review of data indicating that women taking estrogen and progestin had an elevated rate of breast cancer, heart disease and stroke. The news ran a breaking story, newspapers had it in headlines and it even made the cover of Time magazine. Stop the Hormones!

Of course, once it was apparent that no, it wasn't estrogen causing cancer (more on this in the next chapter) where was the cover story? Where was the retraction? Why didn't they announce to the world they made a mistake? Usually something like this that grabs your attention makes better news and somehow this misinformation has lingered for almost 2 decades. Fortunately, hormones are overcoming their bad rap and more people are becoming educated as to what they actually do and why we need them.

In this chapter we will focus on seven hormones; pregnenolone, DHEA, testosterone, estrogen, progesterone, cortisol, and vitamin D. We've already discussed the hormone insulin at length and it will only be referenced here when needed. This chapter is merely a brief overview of the hormones and these will be discussed in detail in both the menopause and andropause chapters.

There is a lot of confusion over the different terminology used for hormones such as bioidentical, natural, and synthetic. This confusion isn't only with patients; providers often don't know the difference well enough to educate their patients properly. Patients are frequently told there are no studies on bioidentical hormones proving they are effective or safe. This is absolutely not true, there is substantial data supporting the safety and efficacy of bioidentical hormones. Because something may not have been read by a clinician in no way denotes its existence. This will be elaborated upon in the Menopause chapter.

Before educating patients on hormone therapy you need to have good understanding of them yourself. Hormones are chemical messengers excreted from endocrine glands and they travel to other cells that have receptors for the chemical. The effects of the chemicals are to assist and regulate body function and processes. Hormones talk to proper functioning cells and organs. An excess of or deficiency of hormones will have specific consequences.

Bioidentical hormones are those that are produced synthetically, often from a plant base, yet are *identical* in every way to that which is made naturally in the human body. They are the number one used type of hormone for menopause in Europe.

Natural hormones are those naturally occurring. Many commercial products such as progesterone creams say they are "natural" and they very well may be – but natural to a plant or animal not a human. Unfortunately, many women buy over the counter progesterone cream made from yams, yet the human body can't synthesize progesterone from yams. In other words, it's useless.

Premarin, the commercial estrogen product is natural, but natural to a horse, not a human. Premarin is derived from the urine of a pregnant mare. Pre (PREgnant) mar (MARe) in (urINe). A horse has over 20 different kinds of estrogens of which only two humans have. In Premarin, there are 11 kinds of horse estrogen used; meaning that 9 of the estrogens used are *not* human. Premarin is a mixture of 30-plussubstances derived from the urine of pregnant mares. Estradiol, the dominant sex-steroid hormone in woman, accounts for only about 17 percent of Premarin's total content.

The collection of urine from over 750,000 horses is barbaric in nature. A horse that is designed to have near constant activity is confined to a slim stall and attached to a urine collection device for at least 6 months. They don't even have room to turn around. These horses are repeatedly impregnated for the sole purpose of collecting their urine. The makers of Premarin are collecting the urine of horses in the Canada, China, Poland, and Kazakhstan as these are the only places it's permitted to make this synthetic drug.

Synthetic doesn't differentiate between bio-identical and non-bioidentical. Non-bioidentical, synthetic hormones are those that are used for purposes such as birth control pills. They are not of the same molecular structure as human hormones or bioidentical hormones and they don't bind to receptors in the same way. Their role in the body is to mimic biological hormone function, which it does to a degree, but what else does it do? When you look at a molecule of estrogen and a molecule of testosterone, they are nearly the same but with ever so slight differences. How they function in the body, however, is completely different.

Look at the following graphic showing differences between biological, human estrogen (top) compared to the structure of synthetic, non-bioidentical estrogen in the birth control pill Yaz (bottom). With its protective clathrate, the estrogen in Yaz looks like the difference between a snowflake and a nuclear plant. When dealing with synthetic hormones from pharmaceutical companies, keep in mind that similar does not mean identical – in appearance or function.

CHOLESTEROL

Cholesterol

Hormones begin within the matrix of cholesterol. Cholesterol is manufactured in the liver and brain which provides approximately 75-80% of the cholesterol in the body. The remainder is from dietary intake. Decreasing dietary cholesterol rarely lowers overall levels within the body because the liver will produce more if the diet has less, and vice versa. Using a drug, such as a statin to lower cholesterol may have great changes seen on paper (and for a select population) yet what is happening within the body doesn't care at all what is printed on a lab sheet. When cholesterol is blocked you are, in essence, also blocking hormone production. This is evident in men who are started on a statin and very quickly their testosterone tanks. But it isn't just the sex hormones that are hampered, it's also vitamin D. Vitamin D isn't actually a vitamin and it is synthesized in the body as a hormone.

Cholesterol is so important that virtually every cell in our body uses it and a disproportionate amount of our cholesterol (about 25%) is used by the brain (about 2% of our body's weight) to function, so it's apparent that it's vital to brain function! Cholesterol cannot penetrate and pass the blood brain barrier so the brain manufactures its own. With cholesterol blocking drugs the brain is deprived of the amount it needs to control mood, memory, and learning. Those functions are drastically reduced; mental health depends on cholesterol! Cholesterol is one of the most important substances within the body that maintain brain health and its ability to function properly. Multiple studies show that higher cholesterol actually reduces the risk of brain disease while increasing longevity.

Dietary choices do not affect cholesterol production; it can be made from carbohydrate, protein or fat. Because of the grave consequences of low cholesterol in the blood and brain, the body is well equipped to maintain the appropriate levels. Studies show us that limiting cholesterol in the diet does not affect serum cholesterol levels. When you eat less your body produces more. The body is smart, it knows what it needs. If you talk to nutrition scientists, they'll tell you one of the biggest myths they hear when discussing to food and supplements is assuming that something you swallow turns into the same something in your body. That's not how digestion and biochemistry work. Eating cholesterol doesn't make your level increase.

Most of cholesterol in the body makes the protective coating (myelin sheath) on the axons of nerve cells. This helps the nerve impulses in thought, movement and sensation. It's essential for life and health. Is it any wonder that people on statins can develop memory issues and other things like muscle pain?

An updated review in 2009 reviewed and republished a study conducted in 2001 that included over 26,000 participants who were all at risk for dementia and/or Alzheimer's disease showed there is no protection from statins on these brain issues. It was once thought that statins would be preventative for disease related to the memory centers of the brain, this study revealed the opposite. Science Daily quoted the lead author, Bernadette McGuinness,

"From these trials, which contained very large numbers and were the gold standard, it appears that statins given in late life to individuals at risk of vascular disease, do not prevent against dementia."

Beatrice Golomb, M.D., of the department of family and preventive medicine at the University of California, San Diego, stated,

"Regarding statins as preventive medicines, there are a number of individual cases in case reports and case series where cognition is clearly and reproducibly adversely affected by statins."

There are many undisputable reports where cognition is clearly and adversely affected by statin use. Studies show either a negative effect on cognition or a neutral effect, never an improvement or as being preventative.

Side effects of the cholesterol lowering statins include:

- Myalgia (muscle pain)
  - Hormone deficiency
  - Liver function abnormalities
  - Muscle weakness...myositis
  - Rhabdomyolysis; elevated CPK
  - Headaches
  - Difficulty concentrating
  - Abdominal pain; diarrhea and/or constipation
  - Rash
  - Memory loss
  - Dizziness
  - Elevated blood sugar; elevated HbA1C; Type 2 Diabetes

Do you notice in the above list the last entry? Elevated blood sugar, elevated A1c, and type 2 diabetes. Yes, some of the very things that increase your risk for having a cardiac event!

People with low cholesterol are more prone to aggression, depression, cancer, suicide and accidents. What does cholesterol have to do with accidents? Remember, it's needed for brain function. Cholesterol is what fuels neurons and they rely heavily on it for function. It's carried through the blood stream by low density lipoproteins (LDL) that many call the "bad cholesterol". LDL isn't good or bad cholesterol because it isn't cholesterol, it's a lipoprotein. What causes it to be "bad" is when it's oxidized; sugar molecules attach to the LDL and change its shape and it becomes oxidized. This change causes it to be less useful and creates increased free radical production.

Studies have shown the correlation between low cholesterol and decreased brain function, all of which leads to an increase in dementia and other neurological problems.

Brain function includes cognitive function as well as memory and reaction/response. If a quick response is needed to avoid a potentially serious bodily threat it may not be sufficient in the person with lower cholesterol.

Cholesterol is needed to maintain the integrity of the cells, so it's also protective and helps with cellular communication. Studies show that older adults with the lowest serum cholesterol levels have the highest mortality rates. In other words, lowering cholesterol may cause not only a disruption of necessary body function but may also shorten the lifespan.

From cholesterol (and the adrenal glands) comes pregnenolone which contains the building blocks for the production of progesterone and DHEA. In the male body, progesterone counters some of the unwanted effects sometimes seen with excess estrogen. Progesterone converts to estrogen in both the male and female body by way of androstenedione. Some testosterone also aromatizes into estrogen in both males and females.

As you look at the following diagram you can see how vital steroid hormones, including cortisol and the sex hormones, come directly from cholesterol.

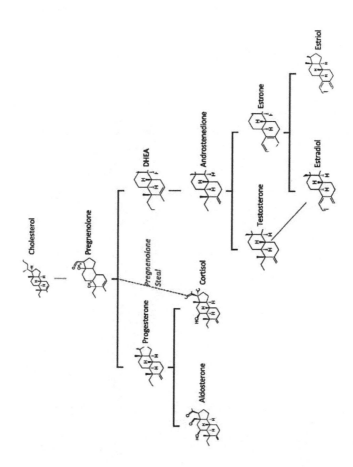

154

PREGNENOLONE

Pregnenolone is the precursor, or starting material, in the production of testosterone, progesterone, cortisol, estrogen and other hormones. Because of this process it's also known as, "the mother of all hormones". It is neuroprotective and has quite powerful effects on aging, memory, mood, sexuality, and sleep. It's produced in the adrenal glands, sex organs, brain and spinal cord. Pregnenolone is found throughout the brain with the highest concentration found in the hippocampus.

A study published in the *Journal of Pharmacological Science* revealed pregnenolone can help with overcoming addictive behaviors and plays an important role in alcohol tolerance levels and withdrawal.

PROGESTERONE

It was once thought that only females with a uterus needed progesterone, yet progesterone receptors are found in both males and females. Aside from reproductive function in the uterus and ovaries, Progesterone receptors are also found in the breast and brain. It plays an important role in a healthy cardiovascular system, bone health and even the central nervous system. This hormone is essential in normal, balanced human physiology. Progesterone in known as the "calming hormone" as it helps with anxiety and also sleep due to its sedative effect by stimulating GABA receptors within the brain. It is also a skin protectant against some androgen effects such a acne and facial/body hair growth.

Other effects of progesterone include:

- Natural antidepressant
- May help libido
- Normalizes blood clotting
- Promotes bone building
- Protects fibrocystic breasts and reduces breast pain

- Promotes sleep
- Reduces hot flashes in peri-menopause and menopause

CORTISOL

Cortisol is also made from pregnenolone and progesterone. When the body detects stress, it makes cortisol a priority. When cortisol levels rise too high it will steal from pregnenolone and halt the production of virtually all these other hormones. DHEA production is slowed to focus on cortisol.

Once upon a time this system was protective, but in today's stress filled world it actually can contribute to many issues such as obesity and type 2 diabetes and their consequential effects. As cortisol rises so does insulin, remember it's one of the non-food events that causes insulin to spike. Reasons for cortisol to rise include waking up in the morning (as does glucose, adrenalin, and insulin – to give you a boost of energy to prepare for the day), not getting enough sleep, exercising, anything that causes acute physical, mental, or emotional stress.

High cortisol has a direct link to increased belly fat. Excess cortisol can decrease thyroid production, specifically T3.

DHEA

We don't know everything DHEA (dehydroepiandrosterone) does, but we do know that it functions as a precursor to male and female sex hormones, including testosterone and estrogen. It's converted from pregnenolone through cholesterol produced in the adrenal glands.

Improvements seen in many things, like strength, libido, illnesses, depression, osteoporosis, etc. can be appreciated with improved DHEA production. This makes sense because it may cause a sub sequential increase in the sex hormones that are produced from it, such as testosterone and estrogens. DHEA 500mg capsules inserted vaginally may help women with sexual dysfunction.

DHEA is synthesized in both adrenal glands and in the brain in particular benefits include:

- Neuroprotection
- Neurite growth
- Heart-antihypertensive
- Anti-Inflammatory–inhibitsIL-6production
- Immune system
- Cognition
- Generation of myelin from oligodendrocytes

ESTROGEN

Contrary to popular belief, estrogen is not the "female hormone" as it is present in both males and females. Estrogen is what we call the group made up of the four major, naturally occurring estrogens in women which are estrone (E1), estradiol (E2), estriol (E3), and estetrol (E4). Estriol is 80% weaker than estradiol. Estradiol is the predominant estrogen during the female reproductive years both in terms of absolute serum levels as well as in terms of estrogenic activity.

It is not, however, the most abundant hormone in the female body during her lifetime. Credit is given to testosterone for that honor. Yes, testosterone is the most abundant, biologically active hormone in the woman throughout the life span. Healthy young women have two to ten times the amount of androgen as they do estrogen.

When we think of estrogen, we typically think of its effects on the reproductive organs, yet estrogen also acts on these systems as well:

- Cardiovascular (women and possibly men)

- Skeletal (men and women)

- Immune (women)

- Gastrointestinal (men and women)

- And neural sites (women)

It is required for:

- Epiphyseal closure of the long bones (men and women)
- Maintenance of bone density and the micro-architecture if bone (men and women)
- Fertility (men and women)

It also plays an important role in the prevention of:

- Premature Coronary Artery Disease (women and possibly men)
- Insulin Resistance (men and women)
- Osteopenia/Osteoporosis (men and women)

Being low or deficient in estrogen can cause many targeted tissues to respond unfavorably and result in clinical disorders. Estrogen helps the body keeping things running smoothly. In the brain, low estrogen in women plays a role in decreased cognition, neural degeneration. Alzheimer's disease risk may also be attributed to low estrogen and hormone replacement therapy may help prevent the disease; this hypothesis is still being studied. It also helps to prevent hot flashes that occur during menopause.

In both men and women with decreased estrogen in the liver and pancreatic tissue, the incidence of metabolic syndrome, obesity and insulin resistance is higher. There is also an increase in inflammatory bowel disease and colon cancer in men with lower estrogen levels; estrogen receptors alpha and beta are both affected by estrogen and studies indicate the balance of estrogen plays an important role in colorectal cancer prevention and treatment.

Estrogen in females is cardioprotective and it's still unclear about being cardioprotective for men. When estrogen levels decline inflammation increases and with that increase the risk for cardiovascular disease goes up. Estrogen plays a role in vasodilation, atherosclerosis, ischemia and hypertension. It is also protective of the reproductive system throughout the lifetime, both before and during the menopausal years. Estrogen also plays an important role (in conjunction with testosterone) in maintaining adequate bone density and maintaining the bone micro-architecture in females as well as males.

Estrogen is a necessary hormone for males as well and issues from being too low, such as weight gain, low libido, fatigue, and osteopenia/osteoporosis are seen when testosterone levels are also too low.

TESTOSTERONE

Testosterone is a pleiotropic hormone which means it has a very wide range of effects in the body. That fact alone shows how imperative it is that levels remain healthy. During childhood, prior to puberty, both males and females have the same, very low level of serum testosterone. Since young children of both sexes have the same levels of testosterone, the notion that it's testosterone which makes the differences in behavior, personality, likes and dislikes between boys and girls, is unfounded. Once they hit puberty testosterone rises in both but obviously climbs higher in males.

Testosterone is known as the "mood stabilizing hormone".

What testosterone does in the body:

- Improves brain function by assisting in the synthesis of neurotransmitter (men and women)
- Improves sleep (men and women)
- Improves sense of well-being and vitality (men and women)

- Essential for libido, arousal, and orgasm (men and women)
- Inhibits fat accumulation (men and women)
- Improves bone density (men and women)
- Anabolic helps to burn fat (men and women)
- Helps to maintain lean muscle mass (men and women)

The brain has many receptors for testosterone and it's clear that the amount can influence how humans think and behave. Sexual thoughts and mood are regulated by hormone levels within the brain which makes sense when you look at sexuality in males verses females as well as mood stabilization with males being more stable during most of the fertile years in this regard.

Muscles cells increase in size and strength in response to higher testosterone levels and fat cells tend to be reduced. Bone density relies on testosterone and estrogen together. The benefits of adequate amounts of testosterone in both sexes are not only numerous but also necessary.

Low testosterone levels are related to

- Hypertension
- Arterial stiffening
- Type 2 diabetes
- Coronary Artery Disease

- Carotid intima media thickness (the innermost layers of the arterial wall)
- Increased cardiovascular mortality
- Increased all-cause mortality
- Increased risk of atrial fibrillation

VITAMIN D

While not technically a vitamin, vitamin D is a secosteroid produced within our body and only naturally obtainable in dietary form from fish and egg yolks. Ultraviolet B (UVB) converts a universally present form of cholesterol, 7-dehydrocholesterol, produced in the skin into D3. After passage through and conversion by way of the liver and kidneys, the end result is a biologically active form of D. Vitamin D functions as a hormone and D1, D2 and D3 are a critical part of the thyroid hormone metabolic pathway.

Vitamin D is an essential substance for health; deficiency of this crucial hormone has been linked to fatigue, weight gain, poor sleep, achy legs (muscle and bone pain), balance issues, fractures, osteoporosis, coronary artery calcification, stroke, congestive heart failure, and accelerated cellular aging.

An inadequate level of vitamin D whether by intake or natural production within the body is associated with osteoporosis and with supplementation the risk of falls in the elderly is reduced by 20%. If the vitamin D regimen includes 700 – 800 IU daily, the risk of hip and vertebral fractures are further reduced and adding calcium. The Recommended Daily Allowance (RDA) for Vit D is 700 mg. When researchers analyzed the study reporting that data, they realized a mathematical error was made and it was missing a 0. It should have been 7,000 not 700. The RDA is the minimum required not for health but for prevention of malnutrition. Supplementation of Vitamin D will be discussed further on.

Increased levels of vitamin D can reduce risks for arthritis of the knee, type 2 diabetes, reduced inflammation, multiple sclerosis, help create a stronger immune system, increased ability to fight some infections such as tuberculosis, and D in ointment form has been approved for psoriasis.

The Women's Health Initiative study demonstrated a 29% reduction in hip fractures after seven years in women who were compliant with supplementation at least 80% of the time. Bone mineral density was increased. The supplement wasn't even very high; they took 400 IU of vitamin D with 1,000 mg of calcium carbonate. By twelve years there was a reduction in vertebral fractures and total cancers including in situ breast cancer and no incidences of invasive breast cancer.

Many lab reference ranges list a low vitamin D level at <30ng/ml; for optimal health and aging the level needs to be at approximately 50 – 70 ng/ml. The reported lower limit of the normal range is totally inadequate for disease prevention. At least a level of 50ng/ml is needed for health correction and 70ng/ml for optimal cellular function. Serum levels below 50ng/ml show an accelerated rate of cellular aging; while achieving the 50 - 70 ng/ml may not slow the aging process beyond normal, but at the least it will return it to a normal aging rate.

Depending on how low the level is, one may need to take a D3 supplement (please avoid the prescription D2, it just doesn't do the job) at 2,000 IUs, 5,000 IUs, or even a 10,000 IU form. Vitamin D3 10,000 IUs with 20mcg of Vitamin K is an excellent way to supplement.

Monitoring serum levels is simple and should be done at least yearly. Yearly intramuscular injections of high dose (50,000 – 500,000 IU) vitamin D3 have been shown to be as effective and often more so than oral supplements due to the non-compliance rate with daily supplements. Oral supplements should be encouraged as the injections may take up to two months to raise the serum levels; I typically use injection for those patients who state they aren't compliant with daily supplements and don't expect to be. D2 injections have been shown to increase fracture rates; stick to D3 whether in oral form or injectable. Toxicity can be an issue but typically at very high doses. As much as 10,000 IU/daily of vitamin D3 is likely to pose no risk of adverse effects.

IMPORTANT!

Always take vitamins A, D, E, and K

with FAT! They are fat soluble so without it you won't absorb much!

5

Menopause

A woman's life stages are measured by fairly predictable stages of reproduction. Reproductive phases are described as beginning after childhood. The first is the reproductive stage, which commences at puberty with completion approximately 30-40 years later. During the earliest time, puberty, the body undergoes numerous hormonal changes which affect fat mass and body shape as well as creating genital, breast and skin changes. The girl begins to menstruate during this time which marks the beginning of womanhood.

The next phase is perimenopause; this is the point in which the menstrual cycle is transitioning from being fertile to a state of infertility. Perimenopause isn't always a black and white issue and is very often quite complex. During this time the woman may experience subtle or dramatic changes; many are not noticeable and many alter daily life. This can be a confusing time for women as the physiological changes are often manifested in emotional or mental changes. Women may not understand why they feel like they do and proclaim, "But nothing has changed"! When, in fact, a lot is changing hormonally and it's just not being recognized for what it is.

Perimenopause can last anywhere from a few weeks to more than ten years; this length of time can lead to the above-mentioned confusion that plagues women. Some of the symptoms related to perimenopause include fatigue, mood changes, inability to lose weight, poor sleep (often the inability to "turn off "thinking" in order to sleep), waking frequently in the night, and being hot for periods of time then cold, especially at night. It also manifests in decreased libido, inability to achieve orgasm, skin changes including adult acne, rogue hairs showing up where women don't want them, and a host of other changes that will be discussed in more detail as we progress. The next reproductive phase is menopause which is the transition into infertility after twelve months of amenorrhea (absence of a monthly menstrual cycle). It's not an official diagnosis until a full twelve months have passed since the last menstrual period (LMP). Once it is established that there has been no menstrual cycle for twelve months the LMP then becomes the Final Menstrual Period (FMP) for documentation purposes.

This can be a very long and frustrating time for many women as it represents one half to one third of their lives. Just when they think they are finished menstruating they have another period. Approximately 90% of women who have gone six months without a period will not have another one, but, then there is the remaining 10%. Eleven months, almost to the finish line, then the process starts all over again. It's almost like playing Monopoly; "Go directly to jail, do not pass go, do not collect $200." Eventually that ends, but the symptoms of actual menopause are just ramping up.

During this critical time in life the woman may experience anywhere from non-existent to profound menopause related symptoms. Some common symptoms of menopause include:

- Hot flashes
- Night Heat/Sweats
- Fatigue
- Loss of libido
- Dry hair
- Dry skin
- Mood changes
- Sleep disturbances
- Urinary tract infections

- Urinary incontinence

- Weight gain

- Depression

Many women become not only depressed but actually suicidal and the hormone changes can destroy their quality of life. There is no need to "suffer through it" as many have been told to do for decades. An important thing to remember is that whether or not you have symptoms there are still medical issues evolving from decreased or deficient hormone levels.

The final phase is the post-menopausal phase characterized by infertility and is often divided into two stages; early stage and late stage.

Premature menopause is defined as menopause which occurs in women equal to or less than forty years of age and is referred to as primary ovarian insufficiency (POI). Regardless of causation, POI is associated with premature osteoporosis, premature cardiovascular disease, and an increased risk of Parkinson's disease. Hormone replacement therapy strongly reduces the risk for premature cardiovascular disease among others.

As we walk through the following related hormones and their role during the different phases of the life span, you will see where and why supplementation is needed and recommended.

TESTOSTERONE, THE LIFE ALTERING HORMONE

Scholarly articles and medical textbooks still refer to testosterone as the "male" hormone even though women also produce it. I've often read that even though women produce testosterone it's in small amounts and estrogen is the main "female" hormone. This is simply incorrect and misleading. As previously mentioned in chapter 4, testosterone is the most abundant, biologically active and available sex hormone circulating in a woman's body throughout her lifetime. In reality, women have between two to ten times more testosterone as they do estrogen! Doesn't it make you wonder why we, as medical professionals, aren't taught this?

Being genetically and biologically similar, both males and females have functioning testosterone receptors (as well as estrogen receptors). Surprisingly, the gene for the testosterone receptor is carried on the X (female) chromosome. Testosterone is also the major substrate for estradiol; the most abundant estrogen. How curriculum continues to falsely represent testosterone in women is confounding. This creates a vastly different hormonal scenario within the female body than reality dictates.

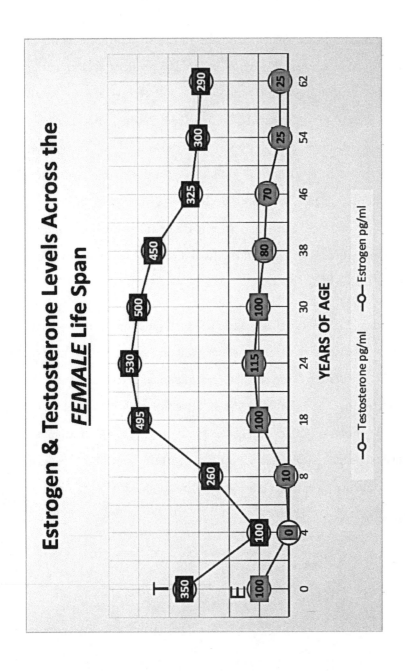

Estrogen & Testosterone Levels Across the _FEMALE_ Life Span

YEARS OF AGE

—O— Testosterone pg/ml   —O— Estrogen pg/ml

Sexual function and libido, despite what is popularly published, is only a very small percentage of the physiological effects that testosterone has in women There are functioning androgen receptors in almost all the tissue in the female body. They are found in the breast, heart, blood vessels, gastrointestinal tract, lung, bronchi, brain, spinal cord, nerves, thyroid, endocrine glands, GI tract, pancreas, kidneys, adrenals, eyes, ears, peripheral nerves, bladder, uterus, ovaries, endocrine glands, vaginal tissue, skin, scalp, hair follicles, bone, bone marrow, synovium, muscle and adipose tissue. All components of metabolic syndrome have been independently associated with low testosterone levels.

Free and Total Testosterone

What is the difference between free and total testosterone levels? The easiest way I have found to explain to patients the difference is this: "Take a box of white ping pong balls, these are each a molecule of testosterone. Throw them out on the floor, that's your total testosterone count. Now take this box of black ping pong balls, these are proteins called sex hormone biding globulin. Throw them onto the floor as well. Every white (testosterone) ball stuck to a black one get rid of; it's no longer useable by the body so it's out of play. The remaining white balls represent your free, unbound, available testosterone. You may have had 160 white ping pong balls at first but after the majority was bound to the black balls you may be left with only 2. Obviously, your free testosterone level will rely heavily on the amount of sex hormone binding globulin you have.

How Does Testosterone Effect Women?

Testosterone peaks in women at approximately age twenty-four. Near twenty-five, the level begins a slow, but steady decline. Women sometimes as young as twenty begin to lose testosterone. Most women 20-40 years of age lose 50% of their testosterone production; this can help you to understand why women feel so much more tired as they get older.

Women see changes in their body near the age of thirty, give or take, and often hear it is a time when their metabolism changed. This change is often attributed to metabolic rate and food, not hormonal changes, but it's the decrease in testosterone that produces much of this change. Weight shifts and a more estrogen body is characterized by fat accumulation in the lower belly, hips, butt and thighs; this is called the gynoid fat distribution.

Testosterone has a reputation among the general public (and some clinicians) as a dangerous hormone that causes men to become aggressive and women to look like men and lose their hair. It's well established that low doses of testosterone restores femininity; it doesn't create masculinity. While too high of doses in women can cause increased masculinity, these high doses are only ethically given to women who are gender transitioning. Higher levels of testosterone, both naturally or supplemented, may increase facial hair growth mildly in some women. Most prefer to deal with that as a separate issue (plucking, shaving, laser treatments, Aldactone (50mg twice daily or 100mg every morning) and continue reaping the benefits of testosterone.

During perimenopause and menopause, testosterone levels are low and can manifest in fatigue, depression, anxiety, irritability, migraines, insomnia, and a general lack of well-being. These are just some of the symptoms of an androgen deficiency which remains widely under treated.

One out of five women have depression as they work through menopause. Micronized progesterone can produce a significant improvement in anxiety and depression for women in peri-menopause, menopause, and pre-menopause if levels are low or they are symptomatic. Mental health is an essential factor in measuring the quality on one's life; this hormonal imbalance should always be corrected before initiating mood altering drugs.

Testosterone is known as the mood stabilizing hormone and creates a physiological harmony with both estrogen and progesterone, helping to keep the body in balance. Young women under thirty are often described as more "stable" in terms of mood and personality, yet over thirty they are sometimes described as moody, unpredictable, and even "crazy". Pre-menstrual syndrome (PMS) is usually more prevalent when testosterone levels fall. Self-descriptors over the age of 30 include depressed, fatigued, out of control, not "myself". This decline happens so slowly that it doesn't register or trigger an "ah ha!" moment defining when the change began.

A typical scenario includes a woman age forty (+/-) who has always been healthy and in great shape. She is active, fit, and mentally healthy. Her body is changing and she doesn't understand why. Her small waist is becoming larger and she is carrying more fat in her middle. She eats a healthy diet but decides to eat less to combat the weight. Her doctor may prescribe a low fat diet for her. She does this and temporarily she experiences some change, but it wasn't significant nor lasting. What explains the temporary, but not permanent change? In part, low, free testosterone levels.

The body has hormone set points and will continue to try to get the body back to those. Her body is going one way when her hormones are fighting to go the other. It's a struggle and she will ultimately not win the battle without correcting the hormones. This can be an extremely frustrating and emotional time for women, nobody wants to suddenly look and feel different.

Remembering that testosterone increases lean mass and decreases fat mass is important because low testosterone does the opposite; increases fat mass and decrease muscle mass. Other changes, such as sagging breasts, face and muscles, can affect their psyche. They live within a society that is now telling them they are no longer beautiful.

By the time a woman is forty most may already benefit from

testosterone replacement therapy; only about 20% of post-menopausal women may not need testosterone supplementation.

Symptoms of low testosterone include:

- Decreased libido/sexual dysfunction
- Difficulty reaching orgasm
- No longer as motivated
- Fatigue
- Insomnia, interrupted sleep, waking between 2 and 3:30 AM not falling back to sleep until 4 or 5 AM. No previous history of insomnia
- Anxiety/Depression
- Lower stamina
- Muscle pain (fibromyalgia)
- Weight gain (especially abdominal)
- Migraines (severity decreases approximately 90% with testosterone levels optimized)
- Increased urinary tract infections
- Urinary incontinence
- Muscles not as strong
- Mental fog
- Multiple aches and pains (arthritis, fibromyalgia)
- Dry eyes
- Autoimmune disease increase

- Feel like I look old

- Don't feel like me anymore

Health risks associated with low testosterone include:

- Osteopenia

- Osteoporosis

- Cardiac disease (10 times more death due to cardiac disease than those with the BrCa genes)

- Breast disease

- Depression

- Obesity

- Type 2 diabetes

- Decreased lean muscle

- Autoimmune disorders (Rheumatoid arthritis, Lupus, Scleroderma, Multiple Sclerosis, Chronic Fatigue, Fibromyalgia, etc.)

- Increase in dental procedures, especially root canals

- Dementia

- Alzheimer's

- Parkinson's

- Sarcopenia (the loss of muscle mass leading to frailty)

- Increased mortality

Blood tests can reveal other changes associated with low testosterone these include:

- Elevated total cholesterol
- Elevated LDL cholesterol
- Elevated triglycerides
- Decreased IGF 1 (growth hormone) less than 150 ng/ml
- Elevated luteinizing hormone (LH) greater than 10-16 u/l (laboratory specific)

Replacing testosterone may normalize levels that are out of the normal range. There are other causes of low testosterone other than the ovaries decreasing production; most of these are common and seen frequently, but may also contribute to more of the very symptoms of low testosterone they are trying to correct.

- Oral contraceptives – birth control pills increase sex hormone binding globulin and decrease free testosterone
- Statins (drugs to lower cholesterol)
- Oral or injected steroids such as prednisone and hydrocortisone
- SSRI's (antidepressants) that increase serotonin and decrease libido
- Antihypertensives (blood pressure medication) that lowers testosterone and decreases sexual response.

- Lupron for endometriosis

- Tamoxifen (drug to treat or prevent breast cancer) it binds to testosterone rendering it biologically unavailable for use.

- Provera (oral, synthetic progestin, a progesterone mimicking drug, increases risk of breast cancer)

There are a few things aside from and in addition to hormone replacement therapy that can influence optimal testosterone levels in women. Supplements including zinc, magnesium, and vitamin D3. Adequate sleep is important in retaining optimal testosterone. Low testosterone causes reduced REM sleep and reduced REM sleep creates lower testosterone cumulating in a vicious cycle.

Diet and exercise do play a role in optimizing testosterone levels. Increasing fats, both saturate and monounsaturated fats will help. Exercise in the form of a combination of cardio, high intensity interval training, and strength training for muscle regulation are very helpful.

Genetics also affects testosterone levels. Inherited genes responsible for regulating amounts of sex hormone binding globulin play a part in free testosterone levels. A "normal" blood testosterone level doesn't indicate receptor site attachment resistance and mitochondrial dysfunction so while there may be plenty circulating in the blood there may be an inadequate amount attached and functioning properly. This is why dosing for symptoms is preferred over dosing for numbers on a lab report. Treat the patient, not the paper! Chasing numbers to please your peers and maybe your patient won't help your patient feel better.

PROGESTERONE

The second hormone to decline is progesterone. This happens around the age of thirty-five. Progesterone, produced in the ovaries, is the calming hormone; progesterone has a sedative effect and helps to resolve hormonally induced insomnia. This is confirmed by poor sleep that returns when stopping exogenous progesterone supplementation. Poor sleep worsens after menopause and is often described as "surface sleeping" where one barely drops into sleep then is awake, repeating until the early morning hours when she finally gets into a deeper sleep not long before having to get up. This, added to the fatigue generated by low testosterone, can lead to a very tired and moody woman. Once the ovaries stop functioning, progesterone is produced by the adrenal glands but the amount is generally much lower leading to symptoms.

Hot flashes and periods of being generally warmer prior to menopause are typically caused by low progesterone. Night heat (hot flashes at night; night sweats) during perimenopause or menopause is also likely related to low progesterone. The term "night heat" is usually recognized by the patient when you mention covers on, covers off, one leg out... I typically get a resounding, "Yes, that's me!"

Progesterone helps to protect the skin from some of the androgenic effects such as acne and facial hair growth. Women in their later thirties often don't understand why they are getting acne when they either never had it or hadn't since their teenage years. This is because, as stated above, at or near their mid-thirty's, progesterone began its decline.

Sleep apnea becomes more common in women after menopause: it is speculated that decreasing progesterone levels are related. Progesterone is a respiratory stimulant and obstructive sleep apnea has been treated successfully with progesterone supplementation.

When progesterone declines estrogen remains higher, creating a larger gap between the two levels. This is referred to as "estrogen dominance" which is nothing more than the avoidance of saying progesterone deficiency. Once there is inadequate progesterone the woman may begin to experience irregular, absent, or heavy periods, bloating, swelling, poor sleep and mood swings.

PMS is more severe when progesterone levels drop and is conventionally treated as a mental health issue and not a physical, hormonal issue. Instead of replacing the deficient hormone, women are given psychiatric drugs.

Successful treatment and resolution of true PMS in a woman of any age is best achieved with optimizing both testosterone and progesterone. Does it make any sense at all to treat the symptoms of PMS with drugs and all their side effects instead of simply replacing what she is deficient in? Does this sound familiar? Treating the symptoms instead of the cause? Think hyperglycemia and hyperinsulinemia…

ESTROGEN

Aging produces the third falling hormone; estrogen. Once estrogen levels decrease dramatically, it triggers menopause and menses cease. With low estrogen women can experience a large number of symptoms. A more comprehensive list follows but here is a small list of issues women may experience:

- Vaginal dryness
- Tearing of vaginal tissue that became thin and fragile
- Dyspareunia (painful intercourse)
- Itching
- Burning
- Bladder spasms
- Increased urinary tract infections
- Urinary incontinence
- Anxiety
- Skin and hair dryness
- Hair shedding
- Worsening insomnia
- Hot flashes
- Greater fatigue

Vulvovaginal atrophy from deficient levels of estrogen affect almost half of women and can lead to a tremendous amount of discomfort. I have treated women who cannot sit on a hard chair due to the significant amount of discomfort. They say it hurts to sit at all, but worse on a hard chair. Intercourse is out of the question. This typically leads to a loss of their sexual satisfaction, loss of intimacy with their partner and it can affect their sleep. This one myriad of changes alone can decrease the woman's quality of life tremendously. Vulvovaginal atrophy is real, it's common, and it hurts.

This happens because the low or absent levels of estrogen cause a thinning and dryness of the vulvar and vaginal tissues. I explain it to patients like this: "Think of the tissue as being like a sponge; the estrogen is like the water that plumps and softens the sponge. Take away the water (estrogen) and sponge becomes dry, flattened and is easier to tear. We need to replenish the tissue with the hormones it is lacking in order restore its health and relieve the discomfort".

Estrogen receptors are most abundant in the vagina although they are located throughout the urogenital system. Testosterone is also found throughout the urogenital system; in the external genitalia you will find the highest density of testosterone. Receptors are located in all the tissue layers of the vagina as well as in the urethra and bladder. Providing testosterone therapy along with estrogen can help to alleviate the urinary symptoms of menopause.

Excess estrogen and testosterone are stored in the fat cells, so during weight loss, when you are breaking those fat cells down, you will have an increased serum level of these hormones. Maybe only until you lose all the weight but possibly longer. So, what does that have to do with bladder leakage? As previously mentioned, adequate hormone levels plump up the tissue like water does a sponge. Now, decrease the hormone and like a sponge, the tissue not only on the vulva but inside around the urethra and bladder structures becomes less healthy.

The urethra sits at an angle that, along with the little muscular valve at the base of the bladder, keeps the urine where it should be until you release it. But when your hormones are deficient and the tissue becomes thinner, changing the angle of the urethra and making the little muscle valve not as tight - voila! You have leakage.

So now that serum hormone levels are increased due to the stored hormone in fat being released into your system, you are in a more natural state of health "down there". You may find this decreasing as the fat loss slows since you will be back to normal production. In some cases, returning the estrogen to adequate levels may actually increase bladder leakage, in that case, a vaginal estrogen cream can help solve or minimize the issue. If young, your body may return to a normal production since weight is no longer a big issue; but if peri or post-menopausal you are likely to see leakage return unless you replenish your estrogen and testosterone, and you need to!

L. Nachtigall noted in a 1999 study that for every 2,000 post-menopausal, untreated women, in any given year, three will have endometrial cancer, six will have breast cancer, eleven will have osteoporosis, 20 will have heart disease and nearly 100% will experience urogenital atrophy.

On physical exam the tissue will appear pale, dry and thin. You may find the introitus (entrance to the vagina) is narrow or constricted. As vulvovaginal atrophy advances, the clitoris may become phimotic (the clitoral hood doesn't completely retract with stimulation) and can lead to discomfort or even pain during sexual activity. Fat pads are lost, primarily seen as a lack of distinction between the labia majora and minora. The elasticity in the vagina is reduced and it may become shorter and narrower and you may see less prominent rugae. The cervix may appear as if it is recessed and more flush with the vaginal wall. Have the patient stand and with your fingers in her vagina have her cough or bear down. If the bladder and/or rectum bulge inward causing the vaginal wall to fall inward they have an obvious prolapse.

Interestingly, women who smoke or have never delivered a baby vaginally may have earlier and more severe symptoms of vulvovaginal atrophy.

Be sure to document the time of onset, the level of associated distress, and the effect it may have on her quality of life. Find out if there is urine leakage when the patient runs, jumps, coughs, sneezes, laughs, or lifts. Is she needing to bend forward or use manual pressure to empty her bladder? This is something that happens so frequently that women often think it's a perfectly normal occurrence.

You also want to include the sexual impact such as intimate partner relationship, level/frequency of sexual activity (women who are more sexually active may report greater discomfort than those who are less sexually active). Make sure to include any history of cancers, age at diagnosis, and if they were hormone dependent. Also, what treatments were/are given. It's important to include age and type of menopause such as spontaneous or surgical, as well as date of LMP or FMP

Differential diagnosis's need to be considered (which is why you need a thorough history). Autoimmune disorders, allergic or inflammatory condition that include vaginitis, contact dermatitis, lichen sclerosis, and even erosive lichen planus. Other possibilities include chronic vaginitis, infections, vaginismus (involuntary clamping down of the vaginal muscles essentially closing it off making penetration not only impossible, but painful. Other differentials include vulvodynia (chronic, painful vulva of unknown etiology), trauma, foreign bodies, chronic pelvic pain, and psychological disorders.

History and physical exam are typically all that is required to make a diagnosis of estrogen deficiency; excluding premature menopause. Asking the right questions can greatly help with forming your diagnosis as is a proper exam, so it's important to investigate the following:

BONES

- Decreased bone mineral density
- Immobility
- Height loss
- Back/joint pain
- Hip/vertebral fractures
- Osteoporosis
- Any fracture after the age of 50 years
- Adjusting the rear view mirror after work (sitting shorter) and readjusting it in the morning (sitting taller).

BREAST

- Breast pain
- Atrophy

MENSTRUAL CYCLE

- Menometrorrhagia (prolonged or excessive bleeding occurs irregularly and more frequently than normal)
- Amenorrhea (absence of menses)

TISSUE

- Night sweats
- Hot flashes
- Collagen loss

- Elasticity loss

- Thinning skin

- Wrinkling skin

- Fat redistribution from hips and thighs to abdomen

GENITOURINARY

- Vaginal atrophy

- Subcutaneous fat loss of labia majora

- Vulvar and vaginal itchiness

- Burning and/or discharge

- Dyspareunia

- Vaginal narrowing/shortening

- Thin, fragile tissue

- Pale tissue

- Easily torn, bleeding skin

- Vaginal pH more alkaline

- Increased rate of vaginal infections

- Urinary frequency, urgency, nocturia

- Dysuria (painful urination)

- Increased number of urinary tract infections

SEXUAL

- Decreased or absent libido

- Dyspareunia

EMOTIONAL

- Depression/altered mood
- Insomnia/other sleep disturbances
- Anxiety
- Irritability
- Foggy thinking/poor memory/dementia
- Decreased quality of life

VARIOUS SIGNS/SYMPTOMS

- Fatigue
- Memory loss
- Dry hair
- Thinning hair
- Sparse eyelashes
- Dry skin
- Thin, wrinkly skin
- Sarcopenia (the degenerative loss of skeletal muscle mass quality, and strength associated with aging. Leads to frailty)

- Accelerated atherosclerosis
- Cardiovascular disease
- Parkinson's disease
- Headaches/migraines
- Heart palpitations
- Macular degeneration
- Increase in immune disorders

6

HORMONE REPLACEMENT THERAPY FOR WOMEN

When possible, I, prefer to treat women preventatively. Hormone replacement therapy can prevent or decrease many issues related to failing health secondary to peri-menopause and menopause. Prevention is key; it's far easier and less expensive to prevent disease than it is to treat or reverse it. Increased quality of life is always paramount, but it's often difficult for women to realize that their quality of life is being impacted by not replacing or optimizing their low and missing hormones. They think what they feel is just the way it is, a natural part of aging. It is, so is going gray and getting wrinkles, but they aren't opposed to dying their hair and getting Botox treatments.

I often hear, "I want to age naturally". So, in other words you are okay with feeling fatigued, having negative skin changes, getting osteoporosis, not being able to think as clearly, poor memory and maybe dementia, heart disease, and becoming frail? Oh and let's not forget that without hormone replacement, earlier death is natural too!

Something to keep in mind; when estrogen is low the follicle stimulating hormone or FSH will rise as the pituitary is telling the ovaries to produce more. If it was "natural" for the body to function with hormone deficiency why does the pituitary continue to demand the ovaries (or medical provider) give it more estrogen?

Years ago women were told to get a different job, deal with it, or to find something that makes them happy. Hormone replacement for the three sex hormones when deficient was taboo, but yet it was okay to replace thyroid hormone when deficient. This bias against women and hormones continues today and has nothing to do with safety and efficacy. Many clinicians are taught to use the lowest dose for the shortest amount of time, yet the North American Menopause Society stated (in their 2017 position statement), "The concept of 'lowest dose for the shortest amount of time' has no basis and may be inadequate or even harmful for some women".

Women who begin hormone replacement therapy live longer with a better quality of life, plain and simple. For those age fifty to fifty-eight show a 43% mortality reduction; under fifty there is a 57% reduction. Incredibly, for women who experienced surgical menopause under the age of fifty and started hormone replacement therapy before age fifty have a 71% decreased rate of mortality!

The biggest obstacle with hormone replacement therapy seems to boil down to a few things. First is the incorrect information given by providers, educators, and the media regarding safety and efficacy. This has gone on since 2002 when the Women's Health Initiative study on hormones was stopped early due to a possible risk of cancer.

The Women's Health Initiative study was planned to span a twenty-year period but stopped ten years short in 2002. It was reported that women on hormone replacement therapy were experiencing an increased rate of breast cancer so continuation of the study would be unethical. The news reported that women on estrogen replacement therapy were at grave risk for breast cancer. It was even on the cover of Time magazine. Medical providers stopped therapy for their patients, and guess what happened? Mortality increased. Breast cancer, however, was not caused by estrogen and once this fact was discovered there was no fanfare, not breaking news stories, no magazine covers. In turn, most medical providers were not even aware of the new findings. So, what were those findings anyway?

The study didn't use bioidentical hormones; it used an oral, conjugated equine estrogen, known as Premarin – remember that is the substance derived from the urine of pregnant horses. It also used a non-bioidentical progestin (notice not progesterone but progestin – two entirely different things) called Provera. Together it was named PremPro. This combination of drugs, specifically the Provera portion is what caused some women to get breast cancer. The rate, however, was minimal.

Understanding that statistical significance is different from medical significance is one thing, however, the increased risk in breast cancer didn't even meet the definition for statistical significance and therefore wasn't considered medically significant.

Consider this; the relative risk of breast cancer in the study was reported to be 1.24, but the risk of breast cancer in night shift workers is 1.51. So why isn't' there a huge campaign to stop women from working at night? Or what about the breast cancer risk in black, American women of using an electric blanket for more than 10 years, at 4.90?

Unfortunately, many physicians and media outlets ignored this fact and treated the information as both statistically and medically significant. Researchers have continued to be vocal in their criticism of the Women's Health Initiative study for its inaccuracy in methods, findings, and conclusions. A fact that *is* significant is that women who have breast cancer actually have a better prognosis if *on* hormone replacement therapy. Imagine that! There is definitely a double standard for reporting bad news versus good news.

In a 1991 study conducted by E.M. Davelaar, it was reported that there was no increase in the incidence of breast cancer during the use of subcutaneous estradiol in 261 women followed from 1972 to Mid 1990's. Less cancers overall than the control group who were on no estrogen replacement therapy. This isn't the only study with these kinds of results and, if so inclined, I urge you to do some research on your own. It's well known higher levels visceral fat are related to increased risks of breast cancer; yet when given exogenous estrogen visceral fat decreases and so does the breast cancer risk.

The first and most often spoken concern among women about hormone replacement is that they will get breast cancer. Little do they know that heart disease kills twice as many more women under forty than breast cancer. It kills roughly four times as many women over the age of sixty than breast cancer and once a woman reaches eighty years old her risk of heart disease related death is seventeen times higher than breast disease. What keeps the heart healthy and helps protect against breast cancer? Fasting and bioidentical hormone replacement therapy. Also, taking Diindolylmethane, known as DIM, (100mg twice daily) is a compound found in cruciferous vegetables including broccoli, cabbage, and cauliflower. It promotes estrogen receptor sensitivity, is an estrogen modulator, and contributes to breast cancer cell apoptosis (cell death).

When you consider hormone replacement therapy, statin therapy, and aspirin therapy, hormone replacement therapy stands alone in being effective in reducing total mortality. Have you heard that before from your medical provider? Have you seen it on magazine covers? Did it dominate the news? Pharmaceutical companies make a lot of money on statin drugs and aspirin but they cannot make money on bioidentical hormones since you cannot patent a naturally occurring substance. Food for thought...

Let's talk about skin and the relationship between skin, estrogen, and inflammation. When estrogen is low the effects on the skin are often apparent. Itchy, drier, thinner and more wrinkled, and changes in the skin's acidity seems to gradually replace the healthier, more supple skin pre-hysterectomy or pre-menopause. As the skin begins to break down, the immune system releases small proteins. These proteins are called cytokines and they signal that there is inflammation in damaged areas of the skin. These miniscule cytokines can leak into the circulatory system and once there is enough of them, they cause inflammation throughout the body. Even if there is only minor changes to the skin, you have to think about the size of the organ; the skin is our largest organ and so with minor changes throughout there are a lot of cytokines released.

Vasomotor symptoms (day/night heat, hot flashes, cold flashes) are reduced with hormone replacement therapy. While these aren't medical issues in and of themselves, they do impact a woman's quality of life and can contribute to medical issues. Cortisol rises approximately 15 minutes after a woman experiences a hot flash. Cortisol, while an essential part of physiology, can be detrimental. Remember that when cortisol rises so does insulin; this essentially stops fat burning.

Being extremely uncomfortable many times per day and night, interrupting sleep, contributing to weight gain, and limiting activities that may bring on more of the same, is unnecessary. There are other drugs, such as Gabapentin and SSRI's that can reduce hot flashes but their efficacy is far less than with bioidentical replacement and have a host of side effects that aren't seen with estrogen replacement.

Using a combination of progesterone and estrogen for reduction of vasomotor symptoms is extremely effective. This covers the different mechanisms for time of day, in terms of hot flashes in daytime versus night heat.

HORMONES AND BONE HEALTH

Using a combination of bioidentical estrogen and testosterone in pellet form is the most effective prevention and treatment of osteopenia and osteoporosis, for both men and women. Pellet therapy shows bone increase by 8.3% in one year compared to 3.5% for estrogen patches and 1-2% per year for oral estrogen.

Nitrogen-containing bisphosphonates, such as alendronate (Fosamax), slow bone resorption by inhibiting osteoclast activity. In other words, it decreases the amount of bone that is broken down and reabsorbed. What it doesn't do is improve bone micro-architecture, but hormone replacement with estrogen and testosterone does. Bone micro-architecture plays an important role in fewer fractures. A DEXA scan only measures density, not micro-architecture.

In postmenopausal women with osteoporosis who are taking a bisphosphonate, there is an increase in bone mineral density over three years' time. Increases of 8.8% at the lumbar spine and 5.9% at the femoral neck. Again, that's an increase in bone growth every THREE years, plus unwanted and potentially dangerous side effects.

The addition of estrogen with the testosterone increases bone sparing therefore increasing bone density even further. Remember what was stated above, pellet therapy shows bone mineral density increase of 8.3% in ONE year vs THREE years for the bisphosphonates... Take a look at the following chart and notice that the control group who did not receive any therapy at all didn't even maintain their bone density; it decreased in that one-year period. This is true for both men and women without differentiation.

Christianson, et al. stated in their 1981 study on bone density,

"There is no direct evidence that the impairment of intestinal calcium aborption observed during menopause and aging can be overcome by calcium supplementation. Moreover, the evidence that calcium supplementation prevents the trabecular bone loss associated with menopause is at best weak...calcium supplementation should therefore not be used as a substitute for sex hormone replacement, which prevents postmenopausal bone loss in most patients and appears to restore intestinal calcium absorption toward normal (Gallagher et al., 1980a)."

Cauley stated in 2015:

"Total estradiol levels, <5 pg/ml were associated with a 2.5-fold increase in hip and vertebral fractures in older women, an association that was independent of age and body weight."

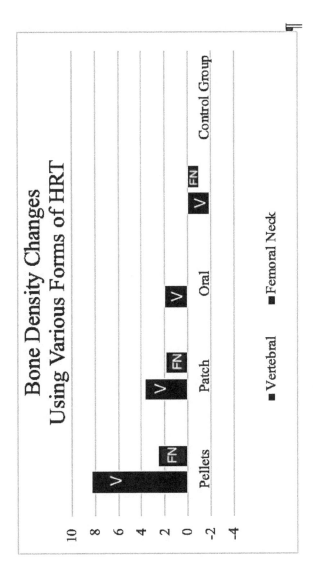

Bone Density Changes Using Various Forms of HRT

This Chart made from information obtained through the following studies: Lindsay, et al, 1976; Christiansen, et al, 1981; Studd, et al, 1990, and Stevenson, et al, 1990.

All of my post-hysterectomy and post-menopausal women not on hormone therapy have total estradiol levels of <5 pg/ml; if any were ever over that I can't remember it, it's very predictable. This is not to say that other women won't have naturally higher levels; it happens.

This is the age of preventative medicine, and to give the appropriate care to patients the provider needs to be aware of these things and act accordingly. If you know that having low sex hormones will increase the risk of osteoporosis, why would you not correct the deficiency? Simply telling your patient to do more exercise, eat calcium rich foods and supplement, is not going to do the trick.

Weight bearing exercise and calcium supplements will not improve bone strength or resistance to fracture in postmenopausal women who do not restore hormone levels with estrogen and testosterone. When considering the very long list of medical maladies associated with hormone deficiency in women, it's baffling why anyone wouldn't choose to replace them.

Upon further investigation you will find that cost is often a factor; most insurance will not cover the costs of hormone replacement. Many claim it's because they aren't FDA (Food and Drug Administration) approved, however, a large amount of drugs are used off label (not FDA approved for a particular use) and insurance companies still cover them. The FDA has approved exogenous testosterone replacement therapy for men with hypogonadal function, but has not approved bioidentical testosterone replacement for women even with documented low levels and symptoms. The only form of testosterone replacement for women that is FDA approved is a synthetic, "EstraTest" which is an oral mixture of methyltestosterone and estrogen, and oral preparations have shown to increase cardiac risks.

It's also been frequently stated that bioidentical hormones created and distributed by compounding pharmacies aren't regulated. This is a misnomer; compounding pharmacies, especially those holding a 503B license and provide patient specific medications are held to higher regulatory standards. These facilities are required to maintain full compliance with current good manufacturing practices. FDA oversight is tremendous for production, sterility, quality and correct dosage.

A note about safety for women starting BHRT greater than ten years post-hysterectomy (with bilateral oophorectomy) or post-menopause. It has been reported that beginning hormone therapy 10 years after menopause increases cardiac risks. It can, although only slightly and that's a temporary effect; the higher risk is only for one year then returns to the baseline risk.

WHAT ABOUT THE PILL?

I once was horrified when a menopausal patient would come to me for hormone help and found that they had been put on birth control pills for "replacement". Now I see it so often it's no longer shocking but still horrifying. It's a quick fix with little thought and even less science to back up its use as a hormonal replacement.

Birth control pills aren't hormone replacement, they are designed to prevent ovulation, ergo pregnancy. They are not the same as bio-identical hormones, so they carry the increased health risks previously discussed regarding non-bioidentical hormones. They also aren't the correct dosage; birth control pills are much higher in dose. Aside from ingredient and dosing differences, there a are a few other things to consider about oral contraception that affects not only the menopausal woman but any woman taking them.

Oral contraceptives have their place and play an important role, without doubt. The problem is they are not designed for short term use so that creates a greater problem; long term use. Why is this a problem? Because you have to look at the issues resulting from long term use that have a great impact on the woman. Oral contraceptives increase the copper level in the body. Zinc levels are reduced and copper and zinc have a very intimate relationship and need balanced in the gastrointestinal tract as well as at a cellular level. The increase in copper can result in an increase in anxiety, insomnia, panic attacks, and hypervigilance. It doesn't take a lot, even a mild increase in copper can result in oxidative stress issues. The increase in copper can also lead to a known side effect of the oral contraceptives; hypertension. Zinc helps to promote a healthy immune system and immune response when called upon. When zinc levels are low the body becomes more vulnerable to infectious dynamics.

It's common knowledge that long-term use of oral contraception depletes vitamin B6 (pyridoxine) which can be a risk factor for estrogen related cancers. B6 is needed for methylation of the estrogen metabolites from their hydroxy form to their methoxy form which makes them less likely to be carcinogenic.

Vitamin B6 and zinc are both needed in adequate amounts to make taurine which is a critical amino acid for body and brain function. A small amount is obtained through foods, however, most of the taurine is produced, synthesized actually, within the body. Taurine serves as a inhibitory neurotransmitter that increases levels of GABA (a neurotransmitter that blocks impulses between nerve cells in the brain) and helps us manage anxiety. To compound the problem, take, for example, the woman on oral contraceptives who is a vegan or a non-dairy eater; the diet is higher in copper and lower in zinc. She has, by way of diet, compounded the problem with oral contraceptive pills by increasing the copper and depleting even more zinc. She is at higher risk of suffering more and worse anxiety, than those who are just vegan or just on oral birth control. Not only that but she also is a prime target for nutritional deficiencies because higher copper and lower zinc in the gut reduce absorption of other nutrients.

If a provider puts a menopausal woman on oral contraceptives this is typically a clear indication that he or she doesn't have current information and training on hormone therapy. This isn't a slight to anyone; I am merely stating that while once an accepted treatment, we have moved beyond that type of drug and dosing to properly address a very treatable condition.

The patient should discontinue the oral contraceptives for a few weeks then have labs run. Once the hormones are balanced the woman feels far better and is more content knowing she is preventing future health issues. Prevention is key; let's do all we can to alleviate current symptoms while preventing future disease states and improving quality of life.

> # IF ON ORAL CONTRACEPTIVES: ALWAYS TAKE ZINC, MAGNESIUM, VITAMIN B6 AND VITAMIN C!

BIO VS NON-BIO EXAMPLE

Bioidentical Estrogen	Nonbioidentical Estrogen
GOOD	*BAD*
↓ ER mediated breast epithelial cell proliferation	↑ Breast cell proliferation,
↓ Estrogen receptor 1 (ER-1) expression	Exhibit estrogen agonist properties in breast tissue
↑ Breast cancer cell apoptosis	↑ Conversion of less powerful estrogens into more powerful estrogens
↓ Breast epithelial cell mitosis	↑ Estrone action
↑ 17-B hydroxysteroid dehydrogenase,	↑ 17-B hydroxysteroid reductase activity

Bioidentical Estrogen	Nonbioidentical Estrogen
continued	*Continued*
↓ Risk of heart attack and stroke	↑ Risk of heart attack and stroke
↓ Risk of atherosclerotic plaques	↓ HDL
↓ VACm-1	↑ Vasospasm
(Vasopressin-activated Ca(2+)-mobilizing, involved in the regulation of signaling)	↑ atherosclerotic plaques
Venous thromboembolism risk not increased	↑ Venous thromboembolism risk
	↑ Insulin resistance

Bioidentical Progesterone	Nonbioidentical Progestin
↓ ER mediated breast epithelial cell proliferation	↑ Breast cell proliferation
↓ Estrogen receptor E1 expression	Exhibit estrogen agonist properties in breast tissue
↑ Breast cell cancer apoptosis	↑ Conversion of less powerful estrogens into more powerful estrogen
↑ Epithelial cell mitosis	↑ Estrone action
↑ 17-B hydroxysteroid dehydrogenase	↑ 17-B hydroxysteroid reductase activity
↓ REDUCES Breast Cancer	↑ CAN INCREASE Breast Cancer

Adapted from Body identical hormone replacement. Post Reprod Health. 2014 Jun;20(2):69-72. Epub 2014 May 22.

WHAT ABOUT OTHER DRUGS?

There are other drugs, such as Gabapentin (Neurontin), that are often prescribed for the treatment of hot flashes. This one really, really bothers me. Gabapentin is a drug for the control of seizures and nerve pain. It *reduces* hot flashes about 60% of the time but it doesn't help with other symptoms of menopause. It also comes with unpleasant side effects. Some of the side effects include dizziness, drowsiness, fatigue, unsteadiness, nausea, diarrhea, constipation, headache, breast swelling, and dry mouth.

Okay, so it helps to reduce hot flashes... does it make sense to add a drug to control one small part of a deficiency? We already learned that hot flashes in peri-menopause are caused by low progesterone and hot flashes post menopause are a combination of low progesterone and low estrogen. Doesn't it make sense to treat the deficiency that is causing the symptoms? Yes, it does. Please don't use gabapentin for symptoms of menopause!

WHAT DOES REPLACEMENT/OPTIMIZATION DO

When deficient, the woman is at increased risk for osteoporosis, type 2 diabetes, dementia, heart disease, breast disease and sarcopenia. She may also experience symptoms, such as fatigue, vasomotor and mood disturbances, decreased libido, painful or absent sex, increased urinary tract infections and an overall lesser quality of life. Replace and optimize those levels and you see a reversal in all of the above and an improved level of well-being. Often the change is monumental.

EFFECTS AND DOSING

Dosing for hormone therapy is configured to meet the patients' needs by considering both the laboratory test results as well as how the patient feels. Levels aren't exact and each patient will have a different level they feel best at and this needs to be priority.

Oral hormone therapy is never recommended (with one exception, progesterone) due to the potential for increased risk of blood clots and stroke. There is also not any oral estrogen or testosterone that is bioidentical, with the possible exception a new oral estrogen drug. Bijuva has recently been released but I haven't researched its details. As a rule, I stay away from those that have a first pass through the liver. Oral non-bioidentical estrogen increases cardiovascular events and it also promotes an increase in sex hormone binding globulin which decreases free testosterone levels.

The one exception for oral use is micronized progesterone. This is patented as Prometrium and because you can't patent a naturally occurring substance the patent was obtained on the unique processing for micronization. This hormone, both generic and brand named, is taken at bedtime due to its sedating properties; it has a remarkable effect on sleep. It may take up to 18 weeks to see a decrease of 80% or more in hot flashes and night heat, but very often does not take nearly that long.

Occasionally someone reports being nauseated with oral micronized progesterone (typically pregnant women taking it for prevention of miscarriage) so I recommend they insert it vaginally. It doesn't provoke nausea but also won't make her sleepy. Progesterone creams also do not help with sleep like the oral micronized progesterone does.

Replacing progesterone has been shown to improve bone density and to decrease hypertension, both very good reasons alone to replace. It increases body temperature resulting in approximately 300 more calories burned each day. It blocks dihydrotestosterone, the androgen that causes acne and rogue hair growth as well as head hair loss. It prevents and treats endometrial cancer, and should always be given when treating with women who have a uterus and are on estrogen therapy. I have encountered more than one physician treating women with estrogen therapy without adding progesterone, a recipe for uterine cancer! It has also been suggested by two studies that progesterone may decrease breast cell growth that is linked to cancer.

I generally prescribe between 100mg and 300mg/day. Post-menopausal always at 300mg/day unless they report feeling more tired early in the day while on it. In that case after they have been on it for a few months, all hormones are optimized, and she still feels more tired, I decrease the dose to 200mg/day or have them take the 200mg orally (for the sleep effect) and 100mg intravaginally as it doesn't cause drowsiness via the vagina. Very often over time they increase it on their own back to the 300mg/day. If headaches are induced back off on the dose and increase slowly. Remind women who are premenopausal that stopping progesterone or missing a dose may cause uterine bleeding and that it's best to be consistent. Progesterone levels are optimal in postmenopausal women at 10 -20 to protect the uterus.

ALLERGY WARNING – Prometrium is made with peanut oil so if there is the possibility of a peanut allergy please use a generic micronized progesterone and speak to the pharmacist about your allergies. Hopefully if this hasn't changed already it **will soon**.

CLINICAL PEARLS

Keep in mind that progesterone and testosterone are breast protectant when considering the use of statin drugs. Statins block cholesterol which decreases testosterone and progesterone, ergo decreased breast protection.

VITAMIN C 500-750mg WILL BOOST PROGESTERONE!

DHEA supplementation is not useful in postmenopausal women or women who have undergone oophorectomy. DHEA is the precursor to testosterone produced in the ovaries which are now either absent or non-functional.

Missing a dose of micronized progesterone may cause menses in post-menopausal women. Be consistent!

IMPORTANT

Obesity = increased estrone in the body. Estrone attaches to the alpha receptors (increases breast cancer risk) and not the beta receptors (breast protective). Therefore, decreased body fat will decrease the risk for breast cancer.

POST-HYSTERECTOMY

Estrogen replacement in hysterectomized women is quite simple and usually without negative effects. Depending on labs, physical exam, or patient report I generally start her with either a 12.5mg, 22mg, or 24mg estradiol pellet. I prefer to start at the lower end and work up, although you will find that some patients clearly need the upper end from the beginning. If the woman appears to have aged rapidly with dry hair and skin, many wrinkles, and has more weight in her middle than hips and thighs, reports hot flashes, night sweats, etc. and has had a hysterectomy, I typically start with 22mg then subsequently back off to 12.5 depending on how she feels.

Estrogen replacement can be a bit trickier in women who are pre-menopausal or post with an intact uterus. Replacing the estrogen can restore health to the uterus and restart menses. This is troublesome for women who have gone years without a period and they typically don't care for restarting. This typically disappears again after a month or two.

Uterine cancer is initially thought of anytime a woman has uterine bleeding after completing twelve months of amenorrhea, often with a rush to get an endometrial biopsy. Estrogen replacement can cause this as well and it's not uncommon at all. For these women I tend to start lower and increase slower; I usually use a 6mg estradiol pellet.

Breast tenderness is common when replenishing estrogen but this will also subside. Many women report decreased or absent symptoms of menopause within 3-5 days, for others it may take as long as a few weeks. Skin changes are a longer process and aren't seen right away. In fact, it happens gradually over time so you probably won't notice a big difference and will forget the dry, sagging skin you once had.

Testosterone replacement dosing, again, is based on lab reports (mainly Free T) and how the patient feels. I typically start women in their later thirties and early forties who are low but not deficient with a 50mg testosterone pellet. They may or may not need estrogen. If near fifty or older, or post-surgical hysterectomy I start with a 100mg testosterone pellet. This is a very common dose, but I do sometimes use 150mg or even 200mg. As previously stated, a "normal" blood testosterone level doesn't indicate receptor site attachment resistance and mitochondrial dysfunction so while there may be plenty circulating in the blood there may be an inadequate amount attached and functioning properly. This is why dosing for symptoms is preferred over dosing for numbers on a lab report. Treat the patient, not the paper! Remember, chasing numbers to please your peers and maybe your patient won't help your patient feel better.

EXAMPLE

Patient X is 54 years old, status post hysterectomy and bilateral oophorectomy 3 years prior. She is complaining of poor sleep, fatigue, daily hot flashes, night heat but not night sweats, weight gain, dry hair and skin. She states she is experiencing some vaginal dryness but not too bad. Intercourse is uncomfortable at times if she doesn't use a lubricant, but not painful. She appears her stated age. Is interested in hormone replacement therapy. After education, lab slip given to test the following:

- TSH
- Free T4
- Free T3
- Total Testosterone
- Free Testosterone
- Progesterone
- FSH & LH
- Estradiol
- Vitamin B12
- Vitamin D
- CBC
- Lipids (not always)
- Fasting insulin
- HgA1c
- HS-CRP

Labs are returned with the following results:

- TSH 3.1 - slightly out of my preferred "good" range of 1.5 – 2.5 (optimal range being 0.5-1.5)

- Free T4 1.0 (optimal being 1.3 – 2.8)

- Free T3 1.6 (good to optimal being 3.2 – 4.2)

- Total Testosterone 32

- Free Testosterone 1.4 (LabCorp method)

- Progesterone <0.1

- FSH 171.9

- Estradiol <5.0

- Vitamin B12 322 (optimal 700 and over)

- Vitamin D 19 (optimal 50-80)

- CBC WNL

- Fasting insulin 12.6 (over 5 is sustained high)

- HgA1c 5.9 (pre-diabetes)

- HS-CRP 3.1 (high risk for cardiac event)

Plan:

Hormone pellets: Testosterone 100mg, Estradiol 22mg, micronized progesterone oral capsules 300mg each night. Recheck labs in 1 month then again just when patient begins to feel any symptoms. I may reduce the estradiol to 12.5 mg after the first time but typically go based on how the patient feels. Remember that blood levels of hormone don't necessarily reflect tissue level. Treat the patient, not the lab slip! Recheck CBC, Total and Free testosterone, estradiol, and FSH approximately one month post pellet insertion. Once the patient starts to notice any return of symptoms, usually 4-6 months after insertion, check labs again. This way you can see the approximate timing of future pellet insertion. Ongoing - check labs yearly.

Vitamin B12 injection weekly (preferred) or oral supplements. Recheck in one year.

Vitamin D3 injection (100,000) followed by oral D3 10,000 IUs + K daily (preferred) or oral D3 5,000 IUs for 3 month – 6 months, then 2,000 IUs ongoing. Recheck in 1 year.

Education on how to reduce CRP, A1c, and insulin – Low refined carbohydrate combined with intermittent fasting. Recheck in one year.

Why am I not addressing the low thyroid function? When testosterone levels are low it's not uncommon to see thyroid function decreased. Once you restore and replenish the testosterone, thyroid levels usually return to normal. If after a few months of hormone replacement, the thyroid levels have not normalized I would start this patient on Armour thyroid. For the patient who has a Free T3 that is low compared to Free T4 I would always use Armour and never Synthroid or levothyroxine as they don't contain T3. If the patient is a poor converter of T4 to T3 it won't do them a bit of good. Free T3 is the most important value in thyroid optimization and a reduced serum Free T3 reduces the resting metabolic rate.

Combination therapy containing T3 and T4 provide superior results than T4 replacement (Synthroid, Levothyroxine) alone. These results include weight loss, energy levels and feelings of well-being.

With Armour, remember it's best to "start low and increase slow", I start with 15mg and increase in increments of 15 mg every 2 weeks until the proper dosage is reached.

SAFER WITH THAN WITHOUT

Breast cancer is the number one health concern reported by women in

general. It isn't, however, the number one health risk. In 2005, 40,000 women died from breast cancer in the United States, that's a lot of women! Makes perfect sense for women to be concerned about getting this terrible disease. During that same year, however, 90,000 women died from stroke and 332,000 women died of heart attacks. Breast cancer is serious, yes, but is not the leading cause of death in women by a long shot. Women are *eight to ten times* more likely to die of a heart attack than breast cancer. In fact, more women die from cardiac disease than all cancers combined.

With cardiac disease being the number one cause of death in women, keep these bits of information in mind:

- Testosterone reduces cardio vascular risk and protects against breast cancer.

- Women with low thyroid levels (Free T3) have a fourfold increase in cardiovascular disease.

- Optimization of Free T3 is critical for lipid control and decreasing cardiovascular risk.

- In the Danish study, after 10 years of randomized treatment, women receiving hormone replacement therapy early after menopause had a significantly reduced risk of mortality, heart failure, or myocardial infarction, without any apparent increase in risk of cancer, venous thromboembolism, or stroke.

- All components of metabolic syndrome have been independently associated with low testosterone levels. Metabolic syndrome leads to cardiovascular disease.

- Testosterone improves insulin resistance.

- Testosterone reduces body fat.

Estrogen is the hormone that many practitioners are afraid to recommend and many women are afraid to use. Of course, the big scare from the Women's Health Initiative is what started this whole fear of hormones and unfortunately the corrections never made the headlines (bad news sells, good news doesn't) so it has continued all these years.

In terms of heart disease, let's take a look at what estrogen does do:

- Increases HDL cholesterol

- Decreased LDL cholesterol

- Relaxes, smooths, dilates blood vessels increasing blood flow
- Soaks up free radicals which are naturally occurring particles in the blood that can cause damage to arteries and other tissue.
- Prevents bone loss and fractures from osteoporosis
- Stroke is decreased in women using hormone replacement versus women not using any replacement (oral estrogen replacement sees an increase in stroke up to 42%, never use oral).
- Does not increase risk of blood clots
- Does not increase risk of breast cancer

CLINICAL PEARLS

Always Balance Estrogen with Progesterone!

(even in hysterectomized women)

- **Natural antidepressant**
- **May help libido**
- **Normalizes blood clotting**
- **Promotes bone building**
- **Protects fibrocystic breasts and reduces breast pain**
- **Promotes sleep**
- **Reduces hot flushes in menopause**

NEVER use oral contraceptives and miscellaneous drugs to treat menopause unless there is an underlying reason!

Estradiol levels should be over 50 and up to around 300, I prefer over 80. I reserve the higher levels for women without a uterus.

7

ANDROPAUSE

Announcements are everywhere for men regarding low T; on the radio, the television, at the gym, in the news… Why is that? Because it's a real issue. The problem with all the radio and television ads is that it causes the appearance of what may be the next latest, greatest fad instead of a true medical issue.

There are many medical providers who treat testosterone deficiency as the real medical issue that it is. On the flip side, there are also providers who prescribe testosterone simply because someone wants it; that is not being ethical or smart. More does not always equate to better.

Speaking of being ethical, neither are, in my opinion, these big box male clinics that charge outrageous prices for something as simple as testosterone replacement therapy. The push to upsell other treatments should make a patient question what the motive behind the "medical care" really is. These businesses often push penis injections of bi-mix and tri-mix, PRP, and other treatments, all of which have their place in medical care, but those are medical options based on the patient's history and current symptoms, not as an "upsell" product. What I have the hardest time with are those that don't tell their young patients that long term exogenous testosterone may render then sterile and offer other options instead.

Low testosterone is a real issue and we are seeing more cases and in younger men all the time. There are numerous theories as to why low T is becoming more common, and one is the exposure to toxins such as pesticides and more estrogens in foods and xenoestrogens from plastics. Genetic causes are typical for those with hypogonadal function but the vast majority of men don't know why they are experiencing symptoms of low T. Some causes of low T can be related to the following:

- Statins (drugs to lower cholesterol)
- Oral or injected steroids such as prednisone and hydrocortisone
- SSRI's (antidepressants) that increase serotonin and decrease libido

- Antihypertensives (blood pressure medication) that lowers testosterone and decreases sexual response.

While you may never know the cause of your or your patient's low testosterone it's important to rule out other medical causes by taking a careful history and evaluation of symptoms along with any other necessary lab tests and physical exam. This may sound a bit odd, but another potential cause of erectile dysfunction is pornography. As the porn watcher sees a higher and higher level of visual stimulation, he can become dependent on it for erections. Always ask your patient and explain to them being brutally honest is what is going to help you help them.

Exploring symptoms is extremely important because most men don't understand that symptoms of low T don't limit themselves to sexual dysfunction and fatigue. There are many other factors to consider, let's take a look at what low T may look like and keep in mind that a man may have one or many of the symptoms, there is no minimum to meet.

A common complaint with many men is a low libido. Again, not all men with low T experience this but many do and for them it's a big deal. The libido encompasses the sexual drive, appetite, urge, and longing. The desire fades from frequent to less frequent and even on to completely absent. This progressive decline in testosterone levels doesn't happen so quickly as to cause alarm but rather gradually and over time. Partners may often notice it first and it can create doubt in the relationship; they may question no longer being desired or even infidelity. These thoughts can be exacerbated by mood changes also noticed and often misinterpreted.

Testosterone is the mood stabilizing hormone and when it's low a man's moods may not be as even keeled as they once were. I've had patients' wives describe them as being, "moody", "bitchy", "PMS-ing", "acting like a woman" and other non-masculine descriptors.

Another common complaint is being fatigued or just tired all the time. I hear many times, "I want to do the things I like to do, that I used to do, but I just don't have the energy to go do it." I also hear, "Every day I plan to go to the gym (play ball, ride my bike, hike, go dancing, etc.) and by the time the work day is over I'm just not feeling up to it and end up on the couch watching TV." Add in some snacks and maybe a beer and call it a day. Some men do say they work out and do things, but are tired much faster than they feel they should be, that their stamina has decreased.

Complaints of "getting a gut", becoming flabby, not being able to build much muscle can also be attributed to low levels of testosterone. When a man's testosterone declines there is more lower belly fat accumulation. Ever notice older, thin men who have a pooching or sagging lower belly? Low T. The high, firm, upper and rounded belly is more typical of high insulin, which, by the way, testosterone helps to decrease. The muscles aren't as dense with low T and building mass becomes harder.

It's important to remember that the heart is a muscle too and just as the biceps, thighs, and glutes become weaker – so does the heart. Keeping all the muscles healthy and strong is important for any man who wants to grow old with vitality. When the muscles begin to shrink and eventually atrophy, this is sarcopenia (the decline of skeletal muscle mass and strength with age) which leads to frailty. It's been described as a common condition in older adults that contributes to functional decline, disability, frailty, and falls. Poor outcomes are more common post-operatively in frail women.

"I want to be old, weak and frail!", said no one. Ever. Being old is a given if lucky enough to live that long; but a body doesn't have to be weak or frail. Low protein has been linked to increased frailty; this makes sense as older people tend to eat less protein rich foods, such as meats.

Another symptom of low T is erectile dysfunction but it's not what you might think. Most men consider erectile dysfunction to mean their penis does not get erect, ever. This, however, is a misnomer; there are varying degrees of erectile dysfunction. This particularly distressing disorder can be from complete absence of an erection to one that just isn't as firm as it once was. It's also quite common for men to state that they have to have constant physical stimulation and/or mental focus in order to remain erect. This is all considered to be erectile dysfunction.

It's important that men understand that being completely honest about their symptoms will get them the most appropriate treatment and meet their unique needs. When you see a patient who has other symptoms but reports no erectile issues, then a month later asks for tadalafil (Cialis) or a similar drug you need to find out what is different now versus during the original interview. Often, they just didn't want to admit they were having difficulty with erections. Help them to build that trust and reinforce the need to be completely transparent about any issues they are having.

As a practitioner you can't always assume erectile problems are related to hormonal deficiency. There could be a medication he is taking, partner issues, stress, performance anxiety, or any number of other health and non-health related possibilities. If you are the practitioner, ask pertinent question regarding other areas of life, talk to your patient, be patient, allow him to express himself in a non-rushed, relaxed atmosphere. If you are the patient, consider this to be a very important discussion with your provider. Finding the correct cause of the issue means you can treat correctly. It's pointless to think one treatment will fix a problem that has deeper roots. It may take a combination of things to get you where you feel your best; be upfront and honest so you can receive comprehensive care with the most optimal outcome.

WHAT HAPPENS (PHYSICALLY) TO THE MALE BODY WITH LOW T?

The human body has many sources of fuel with hormones being a major source. Many of the signs and symptoms for low T in men are the same as for women so much of the same information in the Menopause section will be seen here as well. When a man's testosterone is low, he may experience any or all of the following:

- Decreased libido/sexual dysfunction
- Decreased ejaculate volume
- Difficulty reaching orgasm
- Less intense orgasms (often due to low estrogen)
- No longer as motivated
- Fatigued
- Insomnia, interrupted sleep, waking between 2 and 3:30 AM not falling back to sleep until 4 or 5 AM. No previous history of insomnia
- Lower stamina
- Anxiety/depression
- Muscle pain (fibromyalgia)
- Weight gain (especially abdominal)
- Migraines
- Muscles not as strong
- Mental fog
- Multiple aches and pains (arthritis, fibromyalgia)

- Dry eyes

- Autoimmune disease increase

- Feel like I look old

- Don't feel like me anymore

Health risks associated with low testosterone include:

- Osteopenia

- Osteoporosis

- Cardiac disease

- Depression

- Obesity

- Type 2 diabetes

- Decreased lean muscle

- Autoimmune disorders (Rheumatoid arthritis, Lupus, Scleroderma, Multiple Sclerosis, Chronic Fatigue, Fibromyalgia, etc.)

- Increase in dental procedures, especially root canals

- Dementia

- Alzheimer's

- Parkinson's

- Sarcopenia (the loss of muscle mass leading to frailty)

- Increased mortality

Blood tests can reveal other changes associated with low testosterone these include:

- Elevated total cholesterol

- Elevated LDL cholesterol

- Elevated triglycerides

- Decreased IGF 1 (growth hormone) less than 150 ng/ml

- Elevated luteinizing hormone (LH) greater than 10-16 u/l (laboratory specific)

Replacing testosterone may normalize and optimize levels that are out of the normal range correcting many of the preceding issues.

OSTEOPOROSIS IN MEN?

Do men really get osteoporosis? Yes, they certainly do! Having low testosterone levels leads to secondary osteoporosis in men. Up to 20% of men who have symptomatic, pathologic, vertebral fractures and as many as 50% of men who experience hip fractures are found to be in a hypogonadal state. In a study exploring hypogonadism and osteoporosis, it revealed testosterone replacement was associated with an average of a 39% increase in bone density during that first year. Bone density continued to increase, eventually falling into the normal range which is where it remained throughout the remainder of the study.

While it's true that the risk of hip fracture isn't as in men as it is women, men are twice as likely to die after experiencing one. Typically, estrogen is low in men who have low T; this contributes to osteoporosis due to the mechanism of action of estrogen on bone. Osteoclast (breakdown) and resorption of bone is accelerated with low estrogen, while in reverse, osteoclast activity is diminished with adequate levels of estrogen, thereby keeping bone cells from being reabsorbed as quickly. The notion that men need estrogen blockers while on testosterone therapy is incorrect, they need the conversion of testosterone into estradiol for many physiological functions which is discussed in more detail later in the chapter.

IT SAFE TO REPLACE T?

Safety is a common, and valid concern among both patients and providers. There have been so many myths surrounding the use of testosterone that it's often difficult to know if what we have heard and think is truth or merely speculation. As we discussed in the begging of the book, some things get repeated so many times that we begin to believe it and providers are known to say, "Studies show..." when in actuality they don't show that at all. Let's take a look at some of the myths:

- Testosterone will increase the risk of prostate cancer
- Only older men have low T
- Replacing T will improve sperm count
- Testosterone will increase risk of heart disease
- Testosterone will make my cholesterol shoot up
- Testosterone will cause aggressiveness and rage

- It's illegal to take testosterone

- Testosterone will cause the growth of "man boobs"

- Testosterone therapy will create a ripped body

- Testosterone causes baldness

Let's looks at each of these myths a bit closer.

Myth 1. <u>Testosterone will increase the risk of prostate cancer:</u> No, it won't. Wait! You have heard over and over that it does! You probably weren't told that the whole 'testosterone causes prostate cancer' theory came from a study done by Huggins and Hodges in 1941 and was based on only one man. Yes, one. The men in the study only received testosterone therapy for 14 days. One man eventually had prostate cancer but in no way does that inadequate study show causation. The conclusion that testosterone caused prostatic tumor growth on that one man was based on the use of acid phosphatase which has not been used much due to its erratic results.

Older men with lower testosterone levels are at higher risk for prostate cancer. If most older men don't get replacement therapy, have the lowest levels of serum testosterone *and* the most prostate cancer – how does it make any sense that higher testosterone increases the risk and/or incidence of prostate cancer? It doesn't. I recently had a pre-nursing student ask this very question to her physiology instructor who was teaching them the risks of testosterone and prostate cancer. The instructor had no adequate response.

Multiple studies show that lower testosterone levels are associated with high grade prostate cancer and is also associated with a higher grade at presentation. There are, to date, nineteen studies showing there is no increased risk of prostate cancer with testosterone therapy. It is also known that low T is not protective against prostate cancer. Men utilizing exogenous testosterone have a risk of prostate cancer equal to that of men not receiving exogenous testosterone.

Side note: There are NO studies that show testosterone therapy causes the progression of prostate cancer.

Myth 2. <u>Only older men have low T</u> was addressed in the beginning of the chapter. As previously stated, we are seeing more and more younger men with low serum testosterone levels. I have peers who have had to treat young men, as young as nineteen. My youngest testosterone replacement male is twenty-five years old.

Myth 3. <u>Replacing testosterone will improve sperm count.</u> The pituitary releases Luteinizing Hormone (LH) that cause the Leydig cells to increase production of testosterone and in turn the production of sperm. When exogenous testosterone is in the body at appropriate levels the pituitary can't tell the difference between endogenous (made in the testicles) and exogenous (injected) testosterone. Since the level is adequate the pituitary is not sending the hormone that would result in sperm production. Upon stopping T replacement, the sperm count can improve, however, it doesn't always and any man who wants to preserve his fertility should speak to his provider about alternative therapy, such as HCG and Clomiphene.

Myth 4. <u>Testosterone therapy will increase the risk of heart disease.</u> Low testosterone levels are actually predictive of cardiac disease. Testosterone therapy decreases the dangerous, inflammatory and cardiac risk related visceral fat. The most recent studies indicate there is no connection between testosterone therapy and cardiac disease.

A 2017 study done by Goodale, T. et al. revealed the following:

"Testosterone (T) has a number of important effects on the cardiovascular system. In men, T levels begin to decrease after age 40, and this decrease has been associated with an increase in all-cause mortality and cardiovascular (CV) risk. Low T levels in men may increase their risk of developing coronary artery disease (CAD), metabolic syndrome, and type 2 diabetes. Reduced T levels in men with congestive heart failure (CHF) portends a poor prognosis and is associated with increased mortality. Studies have reported a reduced CV risk with higher endogenous T concentration, improvement of known CV risk factors with T therapy, and reduced mortality in T-deficient men who underwent T replacement therapy versus untreated men. Testosterone replacement therapy (TRT) has been shown to improve myocardial ischemia in men with CAD, improve exercise capacity in patients with CHF, and improve serum glucose levels, HbA1c, and insulin resistance in men with diabetes and prediabetes.

There are no large long-term, placebo-controlled, randomized clinical trials to provide definitive conclusions about TRT and CV risk. However, there currently is no credible evidence that T therapy increases CV risk and substantial evidence that it does not. In fact, existing data suggests that T therapy may offer CV benefits to men."

Think about these facts regarding testosterone's effects on the heart, with both injections and pellets.

Injected testosterone effects on the heart:

- Increases blood flow
- Decreases inflammation
- May increase clotting factors – yet the American Academy of Urology states that testosterone does not cause blood clots. My preference for having my patients donate blood every few months is based on the old premise of clotting; however, I continue to recommend donation every 3-4 months as more of a health benefit than protection from effects of testosterone. There are no studies that show exogenous testosterone causes blood clots. Polycythemia, "thick blood" occurs in all of those living at high altitudes. Their body manufactures more red blood cells, called "erythrocytosis", this is crucial for people at high altitudes to transport more oxygen throughout the body. People living with COPD also have erythrocytosis.

Testosterone via subcutaneous pellets effects on the cardiovascular system:

- Reduces insulin resistance

- Reduces cholesterol

- Reduces visceral fat

- Reduces coronary artery disease

- Increases blood flow to the coronary arteries even in patients with coronary artery disease

- Decreases plaque in the coronary arteries

- Decreases inflammation in the coronary arteries

Myth 5. <u>Testosterone will make cholesterol levels rise.</u> Oral hormones can increase triglycerides but you already know not to give (or take) oral testosterone, right? Right! Injectable hormones decrease total cholesterol and decrease triglycerides but have no effect on high density lipoproteins (HDL). Pellets, on the other hand, affect all three; they decrease total cholesterol and triglycerides and increase HDL

Myth 6. <u>Testosterone causes aggression or rage.</u> Studies indicate no change in aggressiveness with even supraphysiological levels of testosterone. Testosterone may enhance mood and if the man has mood issues such as anger and rage normally this may (or may not) enhance what already exists. Normal human dosing does not cause aggression or rage.

Myth 7. <u>Testosterone is illegal to use.</u> As long as proper credentials and procedures are used for prescribing and ordering, usage of testosterone is not illegal. Testosterone is currently a controlled substance that requires an ordering provider to be in possession of a current, unrestricted license issued by the Drug Enforcement Agency (DEA). Ordering testosterone online, obtaining from a friend, or even from a pharmacist or chemist with a side job of dispensing privately for cash is illegal and dangerous. Always use a provider with proper training and licensure. You have the right to see evidence of both.

Myth 7. <u>Testosterone will make you grow "man boobs".</u> Testosterone may rarely, but generally does not, cause gynecomastia (man boobs). This is more typical with low body levels of testosterone. Men have estrogen receptors in the breast tissue just as women do, and higher levels of estrogen could have an association with gynecomastia. Because of the enzyme aromatase, some testosterone is converted into estrogen which is often to blame for this issue. Think about this; statins decrease testosterone yet gynecomastia is seen in men on statin therapy.

There are many reasons why a man may develop gynecomastia. If testosterone is suspected you can decrease the dosage and see if there are changes. I do not recommend using estrogen blockers as there is no evidence to support this action and estrogen is necessary for maintaining proper bone health.

Myth 8. <u>Testosterone will give you a ripped body.</u> No, it wont. a healthy diet and intense exercise will lead to a ripped body. Testosterone can help improve your muscle development, decrease fat, and improve your stamina for exercise but the rest is up to you.

Myth 9. <u>Testosterone causes baldness.</u> No, testosterone does not cause baldness. The hormone responsible for hair loss is called dihydrotestosterone (DHT) which is an androgen produced as a byproduct of testosterone. If you're genetically inclined to experience to hair loss, DHT can bind to receptors in your hair follicles and cause them to wither and eventually die. This process can eventually lead to a complete absence of scalp hair growth. Your genetics will determine if DHT is going to bind or not.

The benefits of testosterone in terms of mental health, mood, cognition, bone density, and pain control should not be overlooked.

ARE ESTROGEN BLOCKERS NECESSARY?

What constitutes a healthy estradiol level in a male on hormone replacement therapy is controversial, although according to scientific studies, basically all of them, it shouldn't be. I see many patients who come to me already on testosterone therapy and were automatically put on an aromatase inhibitor (estrogen blocker) at initiation of therapy. I have to wonder, what did the practitioner learn that would indicate the need for an estrogen blocker when starting therapy? Young men have estrogen in the 75 -100 range on average, so why do we want disproportionately low estrogen for men in their 40's, 50's and beyond? Do we give aromatase inhibitors to young men since their natural level of estrogen is so high? Breast tissue fat in men is typically a problem of more visceral and subcutaneous fat due to higher insulin levels, not high estrogen. Blocking the estrogen doesn't make the gynecomastia, or "man boobs", disappear; lower estrogen can actually make them appear bigger because inhibiting estrogen increases subcutaneous fat. There is also a genetic component to gynecomastia that can help determine whether a man is going to be affected or not.

There are other causes of gynecomastia which include, aromatase inhibitors (!), statin drugs (by decreasing cholesterol you decrease testosterone and increase visceral fat and insulin resistance, which is why a large percentage of statin users become diabetic), antipsychotics, and androgen deprivation therapy, like Lupron, which is still used by some oncologists and urologists to treat prostate cancer. Many are now adding estrogen (a patch is great) to relieve these men of the many side effects of blocking the testosterone. They feel better, their cognitive abilities return, they no longer have hot flashes and sleep issues. The aromatization of the testosterone into estradiol is very effective in treating the cancer patient and improving their quality of life. Estradiol has an apoptotic effect on cancer cells, isn't this what we want? Yes! Higher doses of estrogen will also lower the PSA.

Past studies were thought to show high estrogen may be a factor in cardiac events, however, they also show those same men had low testosterone – which is a known cardiac risk factor. Remember, association isn't causation and this is a good example.

The body has a balance that is naturally calculated, I agree that adding exogenous testosterone may disrupt the natural balance and we *might* (rarely) need to assist with it, but the natural balance doesn't include an estrogen level of 7! Even the arbitrary 20-30 range for safety is not just odd, but incorrect. Yes, those men with higher or lower levels than the 20-30 had a high rate of cardiac disease but you have to understand that the men in the study (singular) that concluded estradiol levels over 30 were harmful, also had cardiac disease, high triglycerides, diabetes and other issues. Just because the level of estrogen was high doesn't mean is it the cause of the cardiac disease. In fact, studies (multiple) show when estrogen is given to men the risk of cardiac disease goes down. Estrogen receptors dilate the cardiac vessels, that's a good thing! The 20-30 range business is all about association, not causation.

That's equivalent to saying, "It's the children's fault if all the teachers who went to the same late-night party the night before, fall asleep in class the following day. There were children present in each class where the teacher fell asleep, therefore the assumption can be made that it's the children's fault." But what about the teachers who didn't fall asleep and had children in their classrooms? What about the men with high estrogen who didn't have cardiac disease? Again, association doesn't mean causation.

Far too many medical professionals are inclined to believe estrogen is largely irrelevant. It isn't! Estrogens play a fundamental role in the physiology of the reproductive, cardiovascular, skeletal, memory, and central nervous systems, as well as controlling adipose tissue, inflammation, and it is shown to increase lean muscle mass. In addition, it raises high density lipoprotein (HDL). Estrogen is what also improves orgasmic quality, that alone is often all the information a man needs! Seriously, blocking estrogen to achieve a low level is detrimental in many ways. Estrogen levels are the most powerful hormonal predictors of fracture risk in older men. Blocking estrogen, even in small amounts, significantly increases osteoclast activity leading to bone loss. Estrogen levels below 40pmol/liter in men may be the major cause of osteoporosis in older men. If by using an aromatase inhibitor you lose approximately half the benefit of testosterone, why would you? Decreasing estrogen decreases sexual desire, function, and orgasmic quality, is that what men want? I could be wrong, but I highly doubt it. If having low testosterone and low estrogen put you (or your patient) in the category of the highest risk of mortality, why would you not want to raise *both*?

If you feel an estrogen blocker is necessary due to an uncommon to rare issue like breast tenderness that doesn't resolve on its own over a long period of time, I would suggest going slowly on the anastrozole. Starting at 0.25mg on the day of the injection and titrating up from their if necessary. Often, simply lowering the dose of testosterone may help but may also lower it to the point of not being as effective. Check labs every 4-6 weeks until the issue is resolved. Keep in mind that you are decreasing positive benefits of testosterone and estrogen and increasing risks for negative outcomes.

There are natural aromatase inhibitors that don't create adverse situations. Diindolylmethane, also known as DIM, (100mg twice daily) is a compound found in cruciferous vegetables including broccoli, cabbage, and cauliflower. It has anti-inflammatory and anticancer effects, is also shown to increase bone mass and raise testosterone levels. Celery, an aphrodisiac, is a natural testosterone booster, as strange as it sounds, even smelling it can raise testosterone! Other natural aromatase inhibitors include zinc (which is great for the immune system as well), resveratrol, white button mushrooms n (shiitake), and iodine. There are many other health benefits to the consumption of these items, including anti-inflammatory properties, antiviral and anticancer effects. Losing weight will also increase testosterone. How? When your weight is up your estrogen levels are high, this means your follicle stimulating hormone (FSH) and Luteinizing hormone (LH) go down. Lose weight, estrogen drops, FSH goes up stimulating more testosterone production. All without drugs!

There are side effects associated with the use of aromatase inhibitors that need to be relayed to any patient who doesn't understand that they aren't really necessary (and can cause physiological harm) which include:

247

- Breast swelling
- Breast tenderness
- Breast pain
- Body aches
- Body pain
- Sleep issues including insomnia
- Headache
- Thinning hair
- Fatigue
- Sweating
- Flushing
- Increased fat
- Decreased libido

PROSTATE

Prostate-sensitive antigen, more commonly known as PSA, is a protein produced by normal as well as abnormal or malignant cells in the prostate. For years the level was good if under four and with four being the low end of "high". That has recently been changed to high being 2.5. A high free PSA level is good, greater than 25% is typically not cancer. You want a total PSA to less than 2.5 and a free PSA to be 25% or greater. If the PSA is elevated, the first action is to try a round of Bactrim and retest. Most clinicians only order a PSA, ordering a free PSA in addition will give you more information.

Adequate levels of testosterone decrease the lower urinary tract symptoms known as LUTS. These symptoms include hesitancy, poor and/or intermittent stream, straining, prolonged time to empty the bladder, feeling of incomplete bladder emptying, dribbling, frequency, urgency, urge incontinence, and needing to urinate at night. Adequate levels, especially in combination with adequate estradiol levels, decrease benign prostatic hypertrophy, or BPH, which is an enlarged prostate.

ALL FRANK & NO BEANS

As previously noted, when exogenous testosterone is introduced into the body the pituitary slows down its call for the testicles to produce testosterone. In turn, due to decreased activity, the testicles and scrotum tend to shrink up. This is not an issue for most men; I usually hear, "I don't care" or "That doesn't faze me". Aside from a decreased sperm count this is not an issue as it's mainly cosmetic. HCG (human chorionic gonadotropin) can reduce the "shrinkage" of the testicles if the change in size is bothersome for the man.

OTHER OPTIONS FOR ERECTILE ISSUES

When testosterone therapy isn't effective for erectile issues, but if the patient is feeling better in other areas, there is no need to stop therapy. It may be that the patient simply needs an additional treatment in conjunction with testosterone. There are various options which would, of course, depend on the patient's health status, medications, health history, and lifestyle.

If the patient is on an anti-hypertensive, typically a medication change is the first attempt at correcting erectile issues. If it doesn't work there are a few different options that are typically quite effective for most, but like anything else, individuals will respond differently.

There are systemic drugs, such as tadalafil (Cialis) and sildinifil (Viagra) that can increase and maintain erectile function, but not all men are eligible for this type of treatment nor do all men want a systemic effect. For those who cannot or choose to not take either of those medications there are other options for achieving and maintaining an erection.

Medications such as Bi-Mix (Papaverine plus Phentolamine) and Tri-Mix (Papaverine plus Phentolamine plus Alprostadil) are available as a self-administered, penile injection to be used for episodic intercourse. The injections are relatively painless and can be injected manually with very tiny needles or with an auto-injector.

With regular use, the increased blood flow due to the medication can help improve overall blood flow. This can result in improved erections over time, without continued use of the medication. These injections are easy to do and many men (and their partners) are quite happy with the results.

There are also alternatives to help increase blood flow (and often girth and length) for improved erectile function. Men who have had prostate surgery or have erectile dysfunction from poor blood flow due to vascular disease, can benefit from periodic injections of Platelet Rich Plasma (PRP). These injections are done every few months until function is restored or treatment ceases to yield improvement. These injections involve drawing blood, spinning it down to separate platelet rich plasma, then reinjecting into various areas of the numbed penis with a very small, 31-gauge needle. Use of a penis pump after injections of PRP enhance the blood flow and improve treatment outcomes.

With the variety of treatments, drugs, injectables, implanted pumps, etc. available today to treat erectile issues, there is no reason a man should not be able to engage in intercourse that is satisfying and functional.

8

THYROID

We've discussed some of the key hormones; insulin, vitamin D, leptin, ghrelin, progesterone, testosterone, and estrogen. There is another main player that fits well into our discussion; the thyroid hormone. Thyroid issues can be over looked, however, many practitioners are diligent at testing for issues. Unfortunately, they might not be well educated in what tests are actually needed. If you are a provider keep in mind that not all "associations" or practitioners see eye to eye on thyroid issues. I base my information on the education I have through various conferences, individual physician led teachings and lectures on physiology, individual studies that don't use association as causation, and my own research. I encourage everyone to use appropriate studies; that's where you will find the evidence. Using your own diligent research and judgement to treat your patients is ultimately your call.

Not ordering appropriate testing can lead to a missed diagnosis which means the patient isn't going to improve. Before we get into the appropriate tests to order, and why, let's take a look at what thyroid function is all about physiologically. It can be a confusing process so we'll just take it one step at a time.

Thyroid hormone affects all tissue, all organs, and all body systems; think of it as the gas pedal to the body. It's responsible for temperature, metabolism, energy, protein synthesis, cholesterol, fat and protein breakdown. It also helps to improve cognitive function. Thyroid hormone increases the basal metabolic rate (BMR) through increased chemical reactions that are thermogenic or heat producing reactions. There is also an increased use of oxygen, and an increased use of glucose. Disruption of the thyroid process can have from minimal effects to mental retardation and even death. This process must work efficiently or negative changes will happen. The process for thyroid function can be found within the hypothalamus pituitary thyroid axis or HTP Axis.

The HTP Axis consists of 3 main players, the hypothalamus, pituitary, and the thyroid gland. Each of these have processes that affecting the others so each must function properly. When one or more area isn't performing correctly, it causes the others to behave differently with the end result being that the body isn't functioning at an optimal level.

At the center of the brain, near the pituitary gland, is the hypothalamus. A part of the limbic system, this area is responsible for many functions such as coordinating the autonomic nervous system and pituitary function. Other activities include regulating body temperature, thirst, and hunger, but its main role is to keep the body in a constant state of homeostasis.

The pituitary, also called the hypophysis, is a small, pea sized, double lobed gland that is like the mother-ship of the endocrine system. Its main function is controlling growth and development and regulating the function of all the other endocrine glands. The anterior lobe is what is at play in the hypothalamus-pituitary-thyroid axis. The hypothalamus is responsible for detecting and analyzing serum thyroid hormone levels.

When you put the process together from the hypothalamus to the thyroid gland, the process looks like this:

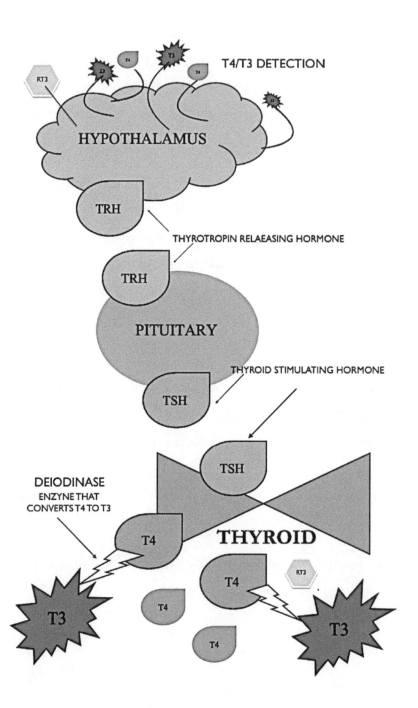

T4/T3 DETECTION

HYPOTHALAMUS

RT3

TRH

THYROTROPIN RELAEASING HORMONE

TRH

PITUITARY

THYROID STIMULATING HORMONE

TSH

TSH

DEIODINASE
ENZYNE THAT
CONVERTS T4 TO T3

T4

THYROID

T4

RT3

T3

T4

T4

T3

As it detects serum levels, the hypothalamus synthesizes and secretes a hormone, called "thyroid releasing hormone" (TRH), to cause either an increase or decrease in production based on a feedback loop (whether it detected high or low levels in the body). TRH is a tripeptide amide which means it is comprised of three amino acids.

The thyroid releasing hormones travel by way of the hypothalamic-hypophysial portal system to the anterior pituitary gland where some of it binds to the pituitary's receptors. For the lay person who may not have been educated on receptor sites; they are kind of like mailboxes. The gland releases the hormone (the mail) and the mail is deposited into the box with the appropriate address. The owner of the mail box is the equivalent of the cell, who then receives the hormone, vitamin, or whatever the intended substance is. If it isn't a match, it's not going to bind to the receptor; it would be like putting the wrong key in a lock or suing the mail analogy, trying to put a square package into a round mail box.

The primary effect of TRH is to triggered the anterior pituitary to release "stimulating hormones" such as thyroid stimulating hormonecommonly known as TSH. TSH is a glycoprotein whose function is to increase the release of preformed thyroid hormone, increase the rate of thyroid hormone production, and cause an increase in size and number of thyroid cells.

TSH then stimulates the thyroid gland by binding to its receptors. The thyroid secretes thyroxine or T4. The gland has thyroid follicles where T4 is produced with the help of iodinated thyroglobulin and other substances, within the colloid. The colloid is a fluid filled, glycoprotein space within the thyrocytes or thyroid follicle.

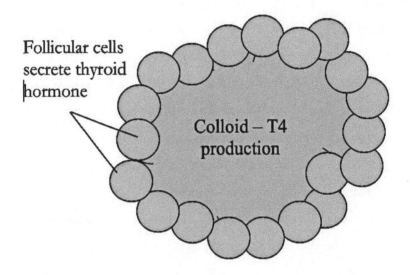

Follicular cells secrete thyroid hormone

Colloid – T4 production

T4 is an inactive form of thyroid hormone; much of it must be converted through a process called de-iodination, into the active thyroid hormone, triiodothyronine, or T3. Most of this conversion happens within the liver although many body tissues can convert T4 to T3. T3 is the thyroid hormone that speaks to every cell in your body; the symptoms of thyroid disfunction begin at the cellular level.

There are a number of factors that can enhance or inhibit the suitable production of T4 and its conversion to T3. For proper production of

T4 there needs to be a nutritional balance; these nutrients consist of iron, iodine, tyrosine, zinc, selenium, vitamins E, B2, B3, B6, C and D. Both zinc and selenium are major players in thyroid health, contributing to proper conversion of T4 to T3. This conversion is dependent upon an enzyme called deiodinase that is largely made up of both zinc and selenium. The body depends on these two nutrients to help maintain proper levels of thyroid hormone. High cortisol can also contribute to low T3 production.

Factors that can impede adequate T4 production are stress, infection, trauma, radiation, medications, fluoride (is an antagonist to iodine), pesticides, mercury, cadmium, lead, and celiac disease.

Influencers of adequate T4 to T3 conversion include, as previously mentioned, selenium and zinc. When these nutrients are low or deficient, there is not proper conversion and they patient will experience symptoms of hypothyroidism even with a normal TSH.

Sometimes the thyroid produces an adequate number of T4 but it just doesn't convert well to T3. One reason is the nutrient deficiency and another is a genetic "poor converter". High insulin levels can impact thyroid function and contribute to poor T4 to T3 conversion. Either way, low T3 equals hypothyroidism. Another situation is that instead of converting the T4 into T3 it gets converted into "Reverse T3" or RT3. What??? Reverse T3?

When the body is experiencing stress, trauma, a low caloric diet, inflammation, toxins, infections, liver or kidney dysfunction, and certain medications (blood pressure medications, diabetic medications, anti-seizure medications, narcotics, and antidepressants) can cause T4 to convert to RT3. RT3 and T3 compete for binding sites on the cells – so, as you can guess, if there is a lot of conversion to RT3 there will not be an adequate amount of T3 interacting with the cells. It's like FedEx and UPS fighting over a mailbox designated for FedEx. UPS packages fit but they are taking up space reserved for FedEx.

The symptoms of hypothyroidism are a reflection of what is happening at the cellular level; to improve cellular reception and function there needs to be an adequate amount of vitamin A, zinc, and exercise.

SIGNS AND SYMPTOMS OF THYROID DYSFUNCTION

Hypothyroid Symptoms (main, there are literally too many to list)

- Course, brittle hair, easily breakable
- Periorbital edema (puffy eyes)
- Facial swelling
- Normal or smaller sized thyroid gland
- Constipation secondary to swelling the gut
- Bradycardia (slow heart rate)
- Cold intolerance

- Weight gain due to using less energy

- Hair loss

- Loss of outer eyebrows

Hyperthyroid Symptoms

- Tachycardia (rapid heart rate)

- Thinning hair

- Hyperreflexia

- Diarrhea secondary to increased peristalsis (increased gut motility)

- Warm, sweaty hands

- Heat intolerance

- Enlarged thyroid or goiter

- Pretibial edema

- Weight loss due to using increased energy

- Exophthalmos (bulging eyes, see follow up explanation)

Subclinical Hypothyroidism is linked with a > 2 fold increase in heart attack risk among women $>$ age 55. Mild thyroid disease is as well established as cardiac risk factor as smoking.

HYPOTHYROIDISM

There are two main types of hypothyroidism, primary and secondary. With primary there are two subtypes, acquired and congenital. One type of primary hypothyroidism, and the most common in the United States, is an autoimmune disease called "Hashimoto's thyroiditis". This happens across all races, but is more prevalent in those with Japanese ancestry.

With Hashimoto's, there is an immune globulin response that is detrimental to the thyroid follicles' epithelial cells and their receptors. These immune globulins attach themselves to the TSH receptors, and like the key that doesn't fit the lock, it doesn't activate the release of T4, instead it destroys the receptors and causes damage and atrophy to the thyroid gland.

The most common form of primary, acquired hypothyroidism worldwide, is called "endemic goiter". This is caused by an iodine deficiency; remember iodide, the ion form of iodine, is a vital element in thyroid function. In many areas of the world, to include the United States, there were low (or absent) levels of iodine in the soil where food was grown. This is because the iodine content of the soil where crops were grown differed geographically. To help with growing number of people affected by goiter, in 1924 the United States began adding potassium iodide to salt, thus making it "iodized".

When the body doesn't get enough iodine to keep it healthy there can be devastating consequences, such as congenital hypothyroidism. Mothers with low iodine during pregnancy give birth to babies with a congenital hypothyroidism, called cretinism. This causes physical deformity, various levels of mental retardation, spastic rigidity, deaf-mutism, and many other symptoms.

For centuries, this devastating disease, Iodine Deficiency Disorder or IDD, was literally destroying the lives of hundreds of children in a remote area of China. The northwestern province of Xinjiang had unusually high rates of congenital hypothyroidism which was destroying the lives and community. This was not new; in the 13th century Marco Polo had documented seeing the people with diminished intelligence, deafness, spasticity and enlarged throats. Fortunately, albeit centuries later, help was on its way.

I had the privilege of getting to know an amazing, multiple prestigious award-winning man, Dr. Robert DeLong. At the time, he was Chief of Pediatric Neurology at Duke University Medical Center in North Carolina, Dr. DeLong is a brilliant neurologist with a distinct and amazing level of social responsibility. Dr. DeLong had seen the devastation of IDD first hand and was determined to help correct the problem. He relayed that he was seeing literally hundreds of affected children. One in ten children had severe IDD, while one in three children showed symptoms of IDD. Those presenting with milder symptoms were described as "slack" and "dull-eyed". Previous, conventional methods of iodine replacement through various trials had failed; but this remarkable man from Indiana had an idea.

In 1992, Dr. DeLong created a system that dripped iodine into the irrigation water that provided iodine to millions of people downstream. Babies were being born without congenital hypothyroidism, more sheep survived, and the communities prospered. After hundreds of years, a cure for endemic cretinism! Dr. Delong essentially prevented more mental retardation in the world than anyone ever has. Iodine, imagine that.

HYPERTHYROIDSIM

Not unlike autoimmune hypothyroidism, hyperthyroidism is also a result of immune globulins attaching to the TSH receptors of the follicular cell. The difference is, however, while these immune globulins damage the cells too, they also trigger them to release thyroid hormone, increase the production of T4, and increase iodine intake. They do this by mimicking a molecule of TSH. This is called Grave's disease.

The immune globulins also attack the fatty tissue behind the eye, by binding with proteins and in turn creates inflammation. This causes the exophthalmos described previously. Exophthalmos isn't a direct result of thyroid gone awry, but more the result of an immunoglobulin attack. Essentially, the thyroid gland dysfunction isn't causing the exophthalmos, but occurs because of the same immunoglobulin affecting the thyroid. This is a good example of association and not causation.

LET'S BREAK IT DOWN

As you can see, thyroid function is unusually complex but relatively straightforward when all systems are working as they should. When they aren't it can be a puzzle; figuring out what pieces aren't fitting needs a little detective work.

Once you understand how the HPT Axis functions, you can more clearly see that there is far more to measuring thyroid function than merely checking the TSH level. Many providers will argue that the TSH is the standard test to determine if the thyroid is "off". And while it *can* tell you the patient is hypothyroid, it doesn't always. Checking only the TSH misses approximately 76% of those with hypothyroidism!

If the patients TSH is high you can give them T4 and their symptoms may or may not go away. They may go away if they were simply low in T4. Now what if you put them on levothyroxine (T4 only) and you now have a normal TSH but the patient doesn't feel any better? Right diagnosis but wrong medication? Correct. Read on.

What about the patient who is symptomatic, yet the TSH is normal or even optimal? Most of these patients will be told, "Well, it's not your thyroid making you feel like that." This is said even when they clearly demonstrate a clinical hypothyroid state.

Upon further testing you may find that while the TSH is normal, the T4 might even be normal, but the free T3 is very low. T3 is what speaks to the cells, and remember that symptoms are derived from what's happening at the cellular level. This patient would be hypothyroid but does not need a drug like levothyroxine. Why? Because levothyroxine is T4 and we have already established the patient has adequate T4. A medication containing T3 is appropriate, such as a desiccated thyroid. Armour Thyroid and Nature-Throid are both popular choices. Remember with desiccated thyroid to start low and go slow. Start at 15 mg every 2 weeks until target dosage is reached. Check T3 levels every month until a stable dose is reached.

Let's look at another situation. Say the patient is symptomatic, has normal TSH, normal T4, and normal T3. Euthyroid? Perhaps, but not necessarily. If you didn't check RT3 you may end up misdiagnosing the patient. If RT3 is high, it will cancel out the T3. Just because the blood has adequate amounts of T3, doesn't mean the cells are getting it. The cells receptors for T3 may have many RT3 molecules hogging the bind. What do you have? That's right, a hypothyroid patient with normal TSH, T4 and T3. What do you give the patient? T3 and measures to reduce stress and cortisol.

You probably can figure out now which lab studies need to be run for a proper diagnosis. History is also important in the investigative process, obtaining a food/diet history may point to possible nutrient deficiencies.

Mostly through a thorough GI and dietary history can you find issues that may be affecting thyroid. Recommended foods that are high in zinc are oysters, red meat, and cheese. Foods that are high in selenium are fish, ham, pork, beef, turkey, chicken, cottage cheese, eggs, brown rice, baked beans, mushrooms, oatmeal, spinach, milk/yogurt, lentils and bananas. Nuts and seeds yes, but we don't absorb as much from plants and it actually can inhibit our absorption of zinc from other sources. So, if you have a vegetarian or vegan patient, they NEED to be on supplements. If your patient has GI issues that decrease absorption like celiac, irritable bowel syndrome, Crohn's disease, etc., they would also need supplementation.

9

PEPTIDE THERAPY

Peptide? What? What the heck is a peptide? A protein is made up of chains of amino acids and a peptide is like a small protein or a short chain. A peptide is made up of 2-50/70 amino acids. It's kind of like the difference between a necklace and a bracelet. A polypeptide is made up of 70 or more amino acids and over 100 is a protein. We have near 300,000 peptides in our body.

Peptides are produced in glands, stomach, intestines and brain. They are found in every cell and tissue of the body and have a variety of crucial functions. Insulin is the most widely recognized peptide hormone. Oxytocin, the love or bonding hormone, is also a peptide.

An appropriate number of peptides is needed to maintain health and homeostasis.

Peptide therapy has a role in regulatory and rejuvenation actions on neuro-endocrine-immune functionality and can also be applied in the treatment of injuries, treat and help prevent chronic disease, and enhance performance. Some of them have a pleiotropic effect, meaning they may be targeting one area and have benefits seen in others.

Let's take a brief look at a few of some of the more common peptide therapies. This is merely a brief overview, enough that you get the idea of what they are and can do. There are many more remarkable peptides available and I encourage you to do some research and exploration.

Peptide therapy is fascinating and may be something you will consider including in your practice. For further reference, there is a great book by Edwin Lee, MD, F.A.C.E who is one of the pioneers in peptide therapy and is a wonderful teacher, eager to spread the word and help others offer this treatment to their patients.

Here are a few peptide examples:

BPC – 157

Pentadecapeptide BPC 157 is made of 15 amino acids and is a partial sequence of the body protection compound (BPC). BPC is isolated from the gastric juice and has been shown to accelerate the healing of wounds such as skin, muscle, bone, tendon, and ligament injuries. It has protective qualities for organs and helps to prevent gastric ulcers. It helps to combat leaky gut, irritable bowel syndrome Crohn's disease, ulcerative colitis and other disorders of the GI system.

People who have suffered from pain and discomfort due to muscle injuries such as tears and sprains report an analgesic affect. It can decrease healing time for burns by increasing blood flow to the affected tissue. Used in combination with platelet rich plasma (PRP) in place of a steroid injections into joints is gaining popularity.

BPC 157 has also anecdotally shown improvement in other areas to include dementia.

Typical dosing for BPC 157 can be done in injections at site of injury subcutaneously. Dosing is 2000mcg/mL, inject 0.15mL daily for 30 days OR Oral 500 mcg capsule, one daily for 90 days. Dosing for human use is less than 10% of study doses.

Semax

Semax is a heptapeptide, neuropeptide that has prolonged neurotropic activity and has shown effective in medical therapy. Pathologies related to brain circulation dysfunction and with different intellectual-amnestic problems of the central nervous system. It is being prescribed for anxiety, memory improvement, ischemic events, stroke, nerve regeneration, ADHD, opioid withdrawal, amyotrophic lateral sclerosis (ALS), Parkinson's, and Alzheimer's disease. It is antithrombotic and fibrinolytic; it also has a gastric protective component.

Semax may improve memory, increase physical performance, and increase the body's adaptation when exposed to high intensity exercise. At higher than average doses it has an analgesic effect.

Typical dosing for Semax nasal spray: 7500mcg/ml, instill two sprays of 0.10ml each, intranasally each day.

Amlexanox

Amlexanox is an anti-inflammatory and anti-allergic compound. It works by inhibiting the release of histamines and leukotrienes. It has been found to produce weight loss and insulin sensitivity. Treating patients with Amlexanox concluded in a statistically significant reduction in hemoglobin A1c and fructosamine. Some patients also saw a reduction in hepatic steatosis.

Typical dosing is one 40mg capsule each day.

CJC 1295

CJC 1295 is a growth hormone secretion stimulator and keeps a steady increase of Human Growth Hormone and IGF-1. It does not increase prolactin and can lead to fat loss.

Typical dosing is 0.10ml injected subcutaneously 5 out of 7 nights at bedtime and with an empty stomach.

Additional Peptides for Therapy

- 3-Disoxy DHEA – reduces aromatase activity, increase
- endogenous testosterone
- Ammonium Tetrathiomolydbate - decreases copper, enhances and decreases resistance to Cisplatin
- Aniracetam – Anxiolytic benefits without sedation
- AOD 9604 + HA -
- AOD 9604
- Dihexa
- DSIP
- Enclomiphene
- Epitalon
- GHK-CU
- IGF-1
- Ipamorelin
- Kisspeptin 10

- LL-37

- Melanotan II

- MK-677

- Peg-MGF

- Pentosan Polysulfate

- Bremelanotide PT 141 (Great for sexual dysfunction in both men and women. Used as needed 30 min prior to sexual activity, shown to have no contraindications and 80% effective in men who don't respond to Sildenafil and Tadalafil)

- SARMS LGD-4033

- Selank

- Tesmorelin

- Tesofensine

- Tetradecylthioacetic Acid

- Thymosin Beta 4

- VIP (Vasoactive Intestinal Peptide)

- Zinc Thymulin

PART

THREE

10

MISCELLANEOUS BITS FOR EVERYONE

There are so many medications, supplements, hormones, and disease do's and don'ts that there is no possible way to know them all. So often we learn about a great piece of information but quickly forget what it was. Hopefully this little reference will be handy in remembering what those little bits of information were all about.

The following is information I find myself telling multiple patients and some or all of it may be of interest to you.

Vitamins

A portion of this information on Vitamin D is purposefully repeated from an earlier chapter on hormones because some readers may only be interested in the weight loss and nutritional topics and may not have read the hormone chapter.

Vitamin D

While not technically a vitamin, vitamin D is a secosteroid produced within our body and only naturally obtainable in dietary form from fish and egg yolks. Ultraviolet B (UVB) converts a universally present form of cholesterol, 7-dehydrocholesterol, produced in the skin into D3. After passage through and conversion by way of the liver and kidneys, the end result is a biologically active form of D. Vitamin D functions as a hormone and D1, D2 and D3 are a critical part of the thyroid hormone metabolic pathway.

Vitamin D is an essential substance for health; deficiency of this crucial hormone has been linked to fatigue, weight gain, poor sleep, achy legs (muscle and bone pain), balance issues, fractures, osteoporosis, coronary artery calcification, stroke, congestive heart failure, and accelerated cellular aging.

An inadequate level of vitamin D whether by intake or natural production within the body is associated with osteoporosis and with supplementation the risk of falls in the elderly is reduced by 20%. If the vitamin D regimen includes 700 – 800 IU daily, the risk of hip and vertebral fractures are further reduced and adding calcium. The

Recommended Daily Allowance (RDA) for Vit D is 700 mg. When researchers analyzed the study reporting that data, they realized a mathematical error was made and it was missing a 0. It should have been 7,000 not 700. The RDA is the minimum required not for health but for prevention of malnutrition. Supplementation of Vitamin D will be discussed further on.

Increased levels of vitamin D can reduce risks for arthritis of the knee, type 2 diabetes, reduced inflammation, multiple sclerosis, help create a stronger immune system, increased ability to fight some infections such as tuberculosis, and D in ointment form has been approved for psoriasis.

The Women's Health Initiative study demonstrated a 29% reduction in hip fractures after seven years in women who were compliant with supplementation at least 80% of the time. Bone mineral density was increased. The supplement wasn't even very high; they took 400 IU of vitamin D with 1,000 mg of calcium carbonate. By twelve years there was a reduction in vertebral fractures and total cancers including in situ breast cancer and no incidences of invasive breast cancer.

Many lab reference ranges list a low vitamin D level at <30ng/ml; for optimal health and aging the level needs to be at approximately 50 – 70 ng/ml. The reported lower limit of the normal range is totally inadequate for disease prevention. At least a level of 50ng/ml is needed for health correction and 70ng/ml for optimal cellular function. Serum levels below 50ng/ml show an accelerated rate of cellular aging; while achieving the 50 - 70 ng/ml may not slow the aging process beyond normal, but at the least it will return it to a normal aging rate.

Depending on how low the level is, one may need to take a D3 supplement (please avoid the prescription D2, it just doesn't do the job) at 2,000 IUs, 5,000 IUs, or even a 10,000 IU form. Vitamin D3 10,000 IUs with 20mcg of Vitamin K is an excellent way to supplement.

Monitoring serum levels is simple and should be done at least yearly. Yearly intramuscular injections of high dose (50,000 – 500,000 IU) vitamin D3 have been shown to be as effective and often more so than oral supplements due to the non-compliance rate with daily supplements. Oral supplements should be encouraged as the injections may take up to two months to raise the serum levels; I typically use injection for those patients who state they aren't compliant with daily supplements and don't expect to be. D2 injections have been shown to increase fracture rates; stick to D3 whether in oral form or injectable. Toxicity can be an issue but typically at very high doses. As much as 10,000 IU/daily of vitamin D3 is likely to pose no risk of adverse effects.

Always take vitamin D with FAT!

B12

Vitamin B12 is also known as Cobalamin. This is a very critical vitamin that can create permanent, irreversible damage when low. Understanding what causes low B12 is something we all should know and be mindful of as it affects far too many people to just pooh pooh the idea of deficiency. In fact, up to 22% of people with type 2 diabetes are deficient in cobalamin.

At the cellular level, low levels of B12 is aging, while improving levels don't reverse aging, it does slow, once again, to a normal rate.

Most of the B12 we get is from meat and is not made within our body. You cannot get B12 from plants; this is why vegetarians and vegans are at high risk for deficiency if they don't supplement daily. We get B12 from meat, eggs, poultry, dairy, and some other meat products. We need B12 to make our red blood cells, nerves, DNA, and many other functions.

Within the lining of the stomach, known as the gastric mucosa, are parietal cells that secrete a glycoprotein called intrinsic factor. This substance is needed for the absorption of vitamin B12, but as the human body ages, intrinsic factor isn't produced in the abundant amount as it was in younger years. 15% to 20% of elderly people are sub clinically deficient in B12 and by sixty years old 48% of men and 52% of women have low hydrochloric acid.

Elderly people, vegetarians, vegans, and those who have had bariatric surgery are at higher risk of deficiency. Pernicious anemia causes low

B12 as well, this is when the body's immune system destroys the parietal cells that secrete the intrinsic factor. There is also a fairly common genetic disorder on rs602662(G;G) that is associated with lower levels of B12. rs602662(A;A) is associated with higher B12 levels. Other issues, such as celiac disease and Crohn's disease can interfere with absorption as well, resulting in a deficiency. Another cause of low B12 is from use of certain medications; one type of mediction are the proton pump inhibitors (PPIs). Some of these are:

- **omeprazole** (Prilosec, Prilosec OTC, Zegerid)

- **lansoprazole** (Prevacid)

- **pantoprazole** (Protonix)

- **rabeprazole** (Aciphex)

- **esomeprazole** (**Nexium**)

- **dexlansoprazole** (Dexilant)

Another medication that lowers Vitamin B12 is Metformin.

Vitamin B12 levels can drop slowly over time or more suddenly.

Symptoms may include:

- strange sensations, numbness, or tingling in the hands, legs, or feet
- difficulty walking (staggering, balance problems)
- Anemia

- a swollen, inflamed tongue
- difficulty thinking and reasoning (cognitive difficulties), or memory loss
- weakness
- fatigue
- Anxiety/Depression

Any older people or those at higher risk for deficiency (previously

listed) should be supplementing either orally or with injections. Any time you notice new forgetfulness in the elderly, loss of balance, weakness, fatigue or even memory issues it's imperative that they have their blood checked for low B12. Any of these neurological issues that persist without treatment for 6 months and more are typically not reversible. Timing is crucial!

Lab tests indicating low B12:

- B12 less than 700 is low, less than 300 is deficient
- MCV greater than 99fL

B3

Also known as niacinamide, vitamin B3 has been used, quite successfully, in patients with osteoarthritis, for decades. A dosage of 1-4 grams, divided 2-3 times daily often results in a decrease in joint deformity arthritis and pain. It is also available as a time released 1500mg pill taken twice daily. Dr. William Kaufman stated,

"The greater the stiffness, the more frequent the doses. Severely crippled arthritic patients needed up to a total of 4,000 mg/day. Divided into 10 doses per day, in one to three months, patients could now get out of their chair, or bed. If continued, they would be able comb their hair and be able to walk upstairs, so they would no longer be prisoners of the house. By the end of about three years' treatment, they would be fully ambulatory, and this was even in the older age groups."

Vitamin C

750mg of vitamin C will help boost progesterone levels

Vitamin A & D – best source is from Cod Liver Oil. Many people are poor converters (genetic, RS7501331 C;T and T;T, and GS239) from beta carotene to vitamin A and should supplement. Symptoms of low vitamin A include poor night vision and when severe can lead to blindness.

Vitamins for Heart Health – According to Dr. Stephen Sinatra, a well-known and highly respected cardiologist, recommends these four supplements and when taken together are the most powerful for heart health:

1. D-Ribose, 5grams twice daily for prevention. D-ribose is a five-carbon sugar, and is one of the components of ATP, the energy molecule the body uses to power all activities.

2. L-carnitine 1000 to 1500 mg daily, in divided doses, on an empty stomach. Up to 3000 mg if you have heart concerns. L-carnitine energizes your heart and protects it from damage.

3. CoQ10, 50 to 150 mg daily. CoQ10 converts fatty acids into energy within the heart. Anyone on a statin drug should ALWAYS take CoQ10!

4. Magnesium 400 to 800 mg daily. Magnesium is a natural calcium channel blocker, a common action of a class of blood pressure medication. Magnesium inhibits clot development and widens and relaxes the blood vessels and arterial walls. It also dilates the arteries reducing blood pressure. Magnesium also helps manage blood sugar!

Other substances for heart health:

-   Alpha-lipoic acid
-   B-vitamins
-   Grape seed
-   L-arginine
-   Marine fish oil

MISCELLANEOUS ISSUES & TIPS

Acne

Niacinamide 4% topical gel used twice daily can greatly decrease acne. A multi-centered, double blind, randomized study of 76 participants with moderately severe inflammatory acne was conducted. After 8 weeks the niacinamide group had a 60% reduction in pustules and a 52% reduction in acne severity, where the clindamycin group saw only a 43% reduction in pustules and 38% reduction in acne severity.

Arthritis

Here is a list of foods to reduce/avoid if you have any kind of arthritis (see B3 above as well) or autoimmune disease:

- Gluten
- Casein
- Safflower oil
- Sunflower oil
- Soy oil
- Corn oils
- Processed meats (lunch meat)
- Syrups & Soft drinks
- Fast food

Arthritis

Niacinimide (Vitamin B3) 1,000 mg three times daily. It may take a few months, but the pain will decrease.

Fibrocystic breasts

Iodine, one drop on breast, alternating daily. Takes time but reduces fibrocystic changes. Also said to help prevent cancer as it kills breast cancer cells.

Hot flashes

Obviously balance hormones first. Second choice is Maca root, 1,000 mg capsules with 4-8 mg of fiber capsule. The fiber helps the estrogen reabsorb in the intestines. Adding DIM can improve estrogen receptor sensitivity.

Inflammation (elevated CRP)

Turmeric (curcumin) helps reduce inflammation in general, for cardiac risk, and is also helpful for pain.

Foods and nutraceuticals that are anti-inflammatories and antioxidants:

- Nuts
- Avocado
- Spinach
- Tart Cherries
- Olive oil
- Orange vegetables
- Pineapple
- Alpha-lipoic acid

- Boswellia (the plant that produces Indian frankincense)
- Carnitine
- CoQ10
- Grape seed
- Marine fish oil
- N-Acetylcysteine

Foods that are pro- inflammatory

If you have a high CRP and other cardiac risks it's imperative that you reduce your intake of these foods:

- Tomatoes
- White potatoes
- Eggplant
- Okra
- Peppers
- Gogi berries
- Tomatillos
- Sorrel
- Gooseberries
- Ground cherries
- Pepino melons (loads of vitamins, protein, iron, copper, calcium, potassium and is a good diuretic!)
- Tobacco
- Paprika

- Cayenne pepper
- Capsicum (bell peppers, all colors)
- Wheat and many other grains
- Sugar
- Meat

Energy boosters
- Ashwagandha
- CoQ10
- Green tea
- Pyrroloquinoline quinone (improves mitochondria function)
- Rhodiola Rosea

Fat oxidation enhancers
- Carnitine
- Conjugated linoleic acid
- Green tea

Glycemic agents and insulin sensitizers
- Cinnamon
- Folate
- Vitamin D

Leg cramps

Soak in a bath of warm water and a cup of Epsom salts. Magnesium is an inorganic salt, often called Epsom. This will also help lower blood pressure, and help with constipation and sleep. Oral magnesium helps as well.

Magnesium and calcium

Needed to buffer the bloods pH – cortisol creates acidic pH.

Melatonin

Increases estrogen receptor function.

Menstrual cramps

Cod Liver Oil mixed with tocopherol. 1 tablespoon twice daily, taper as cramps disappear. For heavy, painful, and clotting menses oral vitamin K, 10-15mg daily for 4-6 months.

Nausea and vomiting

Vitamin K 35mg and Vitamin C 25mg together can eliminate nausea and vomiting, even when it's due to morning sickness.

Nipple sensitivity

Zinc cream (not ointment, it's too thick and messy) twice daily on the nipples can reduce sensitivity. Zinc is a natural estrogen blocker.

PreMenstrual Dysphoric Disorder (PMDD)

Try adding vitamins B6 and E to the treatment regimen.

Preventricular contractions (PVCs)

Magnesium, Co-Q-10 and fish oil

Medicated skin patches

Many people can't use medicated skin patches such as birth control patches, hormonal patches and pain patches due to the skin irritation they experience. Over the counter nasal steroid spray is the answer! Wash and dry the area where you will place the patch. Spray the area with the nasal spray. Allow to dry. Adhere patch as you normally would.

Sprouts

The antioxidant effect of sprouts is highest on day 3 of growth, pick and eat on that day!

Strep throat (frequent)

Don't drink milk! Back aches may also decrease when milk is stopped. If the family has recurring strep, always test everyone; you may have a non-symptomatic carrier. In the absence of a non-symptomatic carrier, swab the pet's noses!

Vaginal dryness, decreased arousal, sensation and orgasm
Intravaginal DHEA improves all those issues!

Zinc superfoods – Oysters, red meat, and cheese!

CONCLUSION

Medicine is an art; sometimes we have to try new things in order to expand our knowledge and see a new picture. As you read this book, I hope you learned something new and perhaps can reach a new level of understanding and experience a new outcome for yourself or your patients.

Moving beyond the outdated information and putting physiology first, my hope is that we can, as a society, overcome the illnesses that have taken over and threaten our lives. If opening others eyes to the reality of the dangers associated with obesity, diabetes, and hormone deficiency helps more people change their lives, we have a fighting chance and winning this battle.

Here's to winning!

ENDNOTES

Foreword

1. Hales CM, Carroll MD, Fryar CD, Ogden CL. Prevalence of obesity among adults and youth: United States, 2015–2016. NCHS data brief, no 288. Hyattsville, MD: National Center for Health Statistics. 2017.
2. World Health Organization [Internet] 2018 Feb 16. Obesity and overweight. Available from: https://www.who.int/newsroom/fact-sheets/detail/obesity-and-overweight. Accessed 2019 Jan 19.
3. Bhupathiraju SN, Hu FB. Epidemiology of Obesity and Diabetes and Their Cardiovascular Complications. *Circ Res.* 2016;118(11):1723-35.

PART ONE

CHAPTER 1

1. Singh AS, Mulder C, Twisk JW, van Mechelen W, Chinapaw MJ. Tracking of childhood overweight into adulthood: a systematic review of the literature. *Obes Rev.* 2008;9(5):474-488.
2. Flegal KM, Kit BK, Orpana H, Graubard BI. Association of all-cause mortality with overweight and obesity using standard body mass index categories: a systematic review and meta-analysis. *JAMA.* 2013;309(1):71-82.
3. National Institutes of Health. Clinical guidelines on the identification, evaluation, and treatment of overweight and obesity in adults—the evidence report. *Obes Res.* 1998;6(suppl 2):51S-209S.
4. Kelly AS, Barlow SE, Rao G, et al; American Heart Association Atherosclerosis, Hypertension, and Obesity in the Young Committee of the Council on Cardiovascular Disease in the Young, Council on Nutrition, Physical Activity and Metabolism,

and Council on Clinical Cardiology. Severe obesity in children and adolescents: identification, associated health risks, and treatment approaches: a scientific statement from the American Heart Association. *Circulation*. 2013;128(15):1689-1712.

5. Schott G, Pachl H, Limbach U, Gundert-Remy U, Ludwig WD, Lieb K. Dtsch Arztebl Int. 2010 Apr; 107(16):279-85. *Epub* 2010 Apr 23.

6. Gigerenzer, G. Helping Doctors and Patients Make Sense of Health Statistics. 2008.

7. Moher D, Shuclz KF, Moher D, et al The CONSORT statement: revised recommendations for improving the quality of reports of parallel-group randomized trials. *The Lancet*. 2001;357(9263):1191-1194. doi:10,1016/s01406736(00)04337-3.

8. Obesity and Metabolism, 12: 83-92. doi:10.1111/j.1463-1326.2010.01275.x

9. Powers M (2005). "Performance-Enhancing Drugs". In Leaver-Dunn D, Houglum J, Harrelson GL. *Principles of Pharmacology for Athletic Trainers*. Slack Incorporated. pp. 331–332. ISBN 1-55642-594-5.

10. Mullington J, Hermann D, Holsboer F, Pollmächer T (September 1996). "Age-dependent suppression of nocturnal growth hormone levels during sleep deprivation". *Neuroendocrinology*. 64 (3): 233–41. doi:10.1159/000127122. PMID 8875441.

11. Wren AM, Small CJ, Ward HL, Murphy KG, Dakin CL, Taheri S, Kennedy AR, Roberts GH, Morgan DG, Ghatei MA, Bloom SR (November 2000). "The novel hypothalamic peptide ghrelin stimulates food intake and growth hormone secretion". *Endocrinology*. 141(11): 4325–8.doi:10.1210/endo.141.11.7873.PMID.11089570.

12. Levine B, Klionsky DJ. Autophagy wins the 2016 Nobel Prize in Physiology or Medicine: Breakthroughs in baker's yeast fuel advances in biomedical research. *Proc Natl Acad Sci U S A*. 2016;114(2):201-205.

13. Matthias B Schulze, Simin Liu, Eric B Rimm, JoAnn E Manson, Walter C Willett, Frank B Hu; Glycemic index, glycemic load, and dietary fiber intake and incidence of type 2 diabetes in younger and middle-aged women, *The American Journal of Clinical Nutrition*, Volume 80, Issue 2, 1 August 2004, Pages 348–356, https://doi.org/10.1093/ajcn/80.2.348

14. Glycemic Index and Dietary Fiber and the Risk of Type 2 Diabetes Allison M. Hodge, Dallas R. English, Kerin O'Dea, Graham G. Giles Diabetes Care Nov 2004, 27 (11) 2701-2706; DOI: 10.2337/diacare.27.11.2701

15. Dietary fiber, glycemic load, and risk of non-insulin-dependent diabetes mellitus in women. Salmerón J, Manson JE, Stampfer MJ, Colditz GA, Wing AL, Willett WC. JAMA. 1997 Feb 12; 277(6):472-7.

16. Dietary fiber, glycemic load, and risk of NIDDM in men. Salmerón J, Ascherio A, Rimm EB, Colditz GA, Spiegelman D, Jenkins DJ, Stampfer MJ, Wing AL, Willett WC. Diabetes Care. 1997 Apr; 20(4):545-50.

17. Modan, Michaela; Halkin H; Almog S; Lusky A; Eshkol A; Shefi M; Shitrit A; Fuchs Z. (March 1985). "Hyperinsulinemia: A link between hypertension obesity and glucose intolerance". J. Clin. Invest. 75 (3): 809–817. doi:10.1172/JCI111776. PMC: 423608. PMID 3884667.

18. Danker, Rache; Chetrit A; Shanik MH; Raz I; Roth J (August 2009). "Basal-stat hyperinsulinemia in healthy normoglycemic adults is predictive of type 2 diabetes over a 24-year follow-up". Diabetes Care 32 (8): 1464–1466. doi:10.2337/dc09-0153. PMC: 2713622. PMID 19435961.

19. Shanik, M.H.; Yuping, X.; Skrha, J.; Danker, R.; Zick, Y.; Roth, J. (2008). "Insulin Resistance and Hyperinsulinemia". Diabetes Care 31 (2): S262–S268. doi:10.2337/dc08-s264.

20. Marinac, Catherine R et al. "Prolonged Nightly Fasting and Breast Cancer Prognosis." *JAMA oncology* vol. 2,8 (2016): 1049-55. doi:10.1001/jamaoncol.2016.0164

PART 2
CHAPTER 4

21. Cholesterol and all-cause mortality in elderly people from the Honolulu Heart Program: a cohort study.

    Lancet. 2001 Aug 4;358(9279):351-5.

22. Total cholesterol and risk of mortality in the oldest old.

    Lancet. 1997 Oct 18;350(9085):1119-23.

23. Center for Advancing Health. "Statins Do Not Help Prevent Alzheimer's Disease, Review Finds." ScienceDaily. ScienceDaily,16April2009www.sciencedaily.com/releases / 2009/04/090415171324.htm.

24. The sigma1 protein as a target for the non-genomic effects of neuro(active)steroids: molecular, physiological, and behavioral aspects. J Pharmacol Sci. 2006 Feb;100(2):93-118. Epub 2006 Feb 11

25. Principi M, Barone M, Pricci M, et al. Ulcerative colitis: from inflammation to cancer. Do estrogen receptors have a role?. *World J Gastroenterol.* 2014;20(33):11496-504.

26. Adiposity, Cardiometabolic Risk, and Vitamin D Status: The Framingham Heart Study Susan Cheng, Joseph M. Massaro, Caroline S. Fox, et al. Diabetes Jan 2010, 59 (1) 242-248; DOI: 10.2337/db09-1011

27. Gupta N, Farooqui KJ, Batra CM, Marwaha RK, Mithal A. Effect of oral versus intramuscular Vitamin D replacement in apparently healthy adults with Vitamin D deficiency. *Indian J Endocrinol Metab.* 2017;21(1):131-136.

28. Kearns MD, Alvarez JA, Tangpricha V. Large, single-dose, oral vitamin D supplementation in adult populations: a systematic review. *Endocr Pract.* 2014;20(4):341-51.

29. Vitamin D toxicity, policy, and science. J Bone Miner Res. 2007 Dec;22 Suppl 2:V64-8. doi: 10.1359/jbmr.07s221.

CHAPTERS 5 & 6

30. Glaser, Rebecca & Dimitrakakis, Constantine. (2013). Testosterone therapy in women: Myths and misconceptions. Maturitas. 74. 10.1016/j.maturitas.2013.01.003. Restoring testosterone levels by adding dehydroepiandrosterone to a drospirenone containing combined oral contraceptive: I. Endocrine effects. *Zimmerman Y, Foidart JM, Pintiaux A, Minon JM, Fauser BC, Cobey K, Coelingh Bennink HJ. Contraception. 2015 Feb; 91(2):127-33. Epub 2014 Nov 13.*

31. Loeser AA. Male hormone in gynaecology and obstetrics and in cancer of the female breast. Obstetrical & Gynecological Survey 1948;3:363–81.

32. Thomas HN, Evans GW, Berlowitz DR, et al. Antihypertensive medications and sexual function in women: baseline data from the SBP intervention trial (SPRINT). *J Hypertens.* 2016;34(6):1224-31.

33. Xuehong Zhang, A. Heather Eliassen, Rulla M. Tamimi, Aditi Hazra, Andrew H. Beck, Myles Brown, Laura C. Collins, Bernard Rosner, Susan E. Hankinson Cancer Epidemiol Biomarkers Prev. Author manuscript; available in PMC 2016 Jun 1. Published in final edited form as: Cancer Epidemiol Biomarkers Prev. 2015 Jun; 24(6): 962–968. Published online 2015 Apr 8. doi: 10.1158/1055-9965.EPI-14-1429

34. Antidepressant-Induced Sexual Dysfunction Associated with Low Serum Free Testosterone Alan J. Cohen, M.D., Private Practice and Assistant Clinic Professor of Psychiatry, UCSF Psychiatry On-Line 1999 revised 10/3/2000

35. Schmidt PJ, Palladino-Negro P, Haq N, Gibson C, Rubinow DR (2006) Pharmacologically-induced hypogonadism and sexual function in healthy young women and men. Endocr Soc Abstr 3:553.

36. Effects of tamoxifen on steroid hormone receptors and hormone concentration and the results of DNA analysis by flow cytometry in endometrial carcinoma. *Nola M, Jukić S, Ilić-Forko J, Babić D, Uzarević B, Petrovecki M, Suchanek E, Skrablin S, Dotlić S, Marusić M. Gynecol Oncol. 1999 Mar; 72(3):331-6*

37. Hadji P, Kauka A, Bauer T, et al: Effects of exemestane and tamoxifen on hormone levels within the Tamoxifen Exemestane Adjuvant Multi- centre (TEAM) Trial: Results of a German substudy. Climacteric 15:460-466, 2012

38. Effect of medroxyprogesterone acetate (Provera) on the metabolism and biological activity of testosterone. *Gordon GG, Southren AL, Tochimoto S, Olivo J, Altman K, Rand J, Lemberger L. J Clin Endocrinol Metab. 1970 Apr; 30(4):449-56.*

39. Night Shift Work Increases the Risks of Multiple Primary Cancers in Women: A Systematic Review and Meta-analysis of 61 Articles XiaYuan, Chenjing Zhu, Manni Wang, Fei Mo, Wei Du and Xuelei Ma Cancer Epidemiol Biomarkers Prev January 1 2018 (27) (1) 25-40; DOI:10.1158/1055-9965.EPI-17-0221

40. Mosekilde L, Hermann AP, Beck-Nielsen H, Charles P, Nielsen SP, Sorensen OH. The Danish Osteoporosis Prevention Study (DOPS): project design and inclusion of 2000 normal perimenopausal women. Maturitas1999;31:207-19.

41. Robarge, Jason, et al. "Electric Blanket Use and Breast Cancer." *Epidemiology*, vol. 15, no. 3, 2004, pp. 375–378.*JSTOR*, www.jstor.org/stable/20485911.

42. Swain, S & Santen, R & Burger, H & Pritchard, K. (1999). Treatment of Estrogen Deficiency Symptoms in Women Surviving Breast Cancer: Part 4: Urogenital Atrophy, Vasomotor

Instability, Sleep Disorders, and Related Symptoms. Oncology (Williston Park, N.Y.). 13. 551-+.

43. The 2017 hormone therapy position statement of the North American Menopause Society. Menopause. 2017;24:728-53

44. Wiersinga, et al.Hormone Research in Pediatrics 2001; 56:74-81

45. Welle, S,L. et al Metabolism, April 1986: 289-291 J. Clinical Endoc and Metabolism 2005 May;90: 2666-2674

46. Shifren JL et al. Transdermal testosterone Therapy in Women with impaired sexual function after oophorectomy. NEJM. 2000 Sep 7;343(10) 682-688

47. Studd, J WW, et al (1990) *Am Journal OB/GYN 163*, 1474-1479

48. Christiansen, C., M.S. Christensen, P. McNair, C. Hagen, K.E. Stocklund, and I. Transbol. 1980. Prevention of early postmenopausal bone loss: controlled 2-year study in 315 normal females. Eur. J. Clin. Invest. 10:273-279. [

49. Christiansen, C., M.S. Christensen, and I. Transbol. 1981. Bone mass in postmenopausal women after withdrawal of oestrogen/gestagen replacement therapy. Lancet 1:459-461.

50. Lindsay R, McPherson SG, Anderson JB, Smith DA. The value of bone density measurements in predicting the risk of developing avascular necrosis following renal transplantation. Calcif Tissue Res. 1976 Aug;21 Suppl:242-6.

51. Eastell R, Barton I, Hannon RA, Chines A, Garnero P, Delmas PD. Relationship of early changes in bone resorption to the reduction in fracture risk with risedronate. *J Bone Miner Res* 2003; **18**: 1051–6.

52. Stevenson JC, Cust MP, Gangar KF, Hillard TC, Lees B, Whitehead MI. Effects of transdermal versus oral hormone replacement therapy on bone density in spine and proximal femur in postmenopausal women. Lancet. 1990 Aug 4;336(8710):265-9.

53. Estrogen and bone health in men and women.

Steroids. 2015 Jul;99(Pt A):11-5. doi: 10.1016/j.steroids.2014.12.010. Epub 2014 Dec 30.

54. Guzick DS, et al. Sex , Hormones and Hysterectomies. N England J of Medicine 2000 Sept 7;343(10) 730-731

55. *Am J Obstet Gynecol*, 2002 Aug; 187(2):289-94; discussion 294-5 ERT does NOT increase either risk of recurrent or death in patients with early breast CA

56. Davelaar EM, Gerretsen G, Relyveld J. [No increase in the incidence of breast carcinoma with subcutaneous administration of estradiol]. Ned Tijdschr Geneeskd.
1991 Apr 6;135(14):613-5. Dutch. PubMed PMID: 2030789.

57. Marttunen MB, et al, A prospective study on women with history of breast CA and with or without ERT, *Maturitas*, 2001 Sept 28;39(3):217-25 Symptomatic pts benefited from ERT without increasing risk of recurrence

58. Body identical hormone replacement. Post Reprod Health. 2014 Jun;20(2):69-72. Epub 2014 May 22.

CHAPTER 7

59. Metter EJ, Conwit R, Tobin J, Fozard JL. Age-associated loss of power and strength in the upper extremities in women and men. J Gerontol A Biol Sci Med Sci. 1997;52:B267–B276.

60. Khera M, Crawford D, Morales A, Salonia A, Morgentaler A. A new era of testosterone and prostate cancer: from physiology to clinical implications. Eur Urol. 2014 Jan;65(1):115-23. doi: 10.1016/j.eururo.2013.08.015. Epub 2013 Aug 16. Review. PubMed PMID: 24011426.

61. Alexander GC, Iyer G, Lucas E, Lin D, Singh S. Cardiovascular Risks of Exogenous Testosterone Use Among Men: A Systematic Review and Meta-Analysis. Am J Med. 2017 Mar;130(3):293-305. doi: 10.1016/j.amjmed. 2016.09.017. Epub 2016 Oct14. Review. PubMed PMID: 27751897

62. Goodale T, Sadhu A, Petak S, Robbins R. Testosterone and the Heart. Methodist Debakey Cardiovasc J. 2017 Apr-Jun;13(2):68-72. doi: 10.14797/mdcj-13-2-68.

63. JCEM 2005;90:6257-62 JAMA. 2009 May 13;301(18):1892-901 J Clin Endocrinol Metab. 2009 Jul;94(7):2482-8 1/28/2 017

64. Low Protein Intake is Associated with Frailty in Older Adults: A Systematic Review and Meta-Analysis of Observational Studies. Coelho-Junior HJ, Rodrigues B., Uchida M, Marzetti E. Nutrients. 2018 Sep 19; 10(9). Epub 2018 Sep 19.

65. Clavell-Hernández J, Wang R. Emerging Evidences in the Long Standing Controversy Regarding Testosterone Replacement Therapy and Cardiovascular Events. World J Mens Health. 2018 May;36(2):92-102. doi: 10.5534/wjmh.17050. Review. PubMed PMID: 29706034; PubMed Central PMCID: PMC5924961

66. Metabolic and behavioral effects of high-dose, exogenous testosterone in healthy men. J Clin Endocrinol Metab. 1994 Aug;79(2):561-7.

67. Metabolic and behavioral effects of high-dose, exogenous testosterone in healthy men. J Clin Endocrinol Metab. 1994 Aug;79(2):561-7.

68. The effects of exogenous testosterone on sexuality and mood of normal men. J Clin Endocrinol Metab. 1992 Dec;75(6):1503-

69. The effects of supraphysiological doses of testosterone on angry behavior in healthy eugonadal men--a clinical research center study. J Clin Endocrinol Metab. 1996 Oct;81(10):3754-8.

70. Statin medications and the risk of gynecomastia. Clin Endocrinol (Oxf). 2018 Oct;89(4):470-473. doi: 10.1111/ cen.13794. Epub 2018 Jul 15.

71. Mauvais-Jarvis, Franck et al. "The role of estrogens in control of energy balance and glucose homeostasis." *Endocrine reviews* vol. 34,3 (2013): 309-38. doi:10.1210/er.2012-1055

72. Long-term effect of testosterone therapy on bone mineral density in hypogonadal men. *Behre HM, Kliesch S, Leifke E, Link TM, Nieschlag E J Clin Endocrinol Metab. 1997 Aug; 82(8):2386-90.*

73. Katz DJ1, Nabulsi O, Tal R, Mulhall JP. BJU Int. 2012 Aug;110(4):573-8. doi: 10.1111/j.1464-410X.2011.10702.x. Epub 2011 Nov 1.

CHAPATER 8

74. Danzi S et al. Potential uses of T3 in treatment of human disease. Clin Cornerstone 2005;7 Suppl 2:S9-15.

75. Bunevicius R et al. Effects of thyroxine as compared with thyroxine plus triiodothyronine in patients with hypothyroidism. N Engl J Med 1999 Feb 11;340(6):424-9

76. Hoang TD et al. Desiccated thyroid extract compared with levothyroxine in treatment of hypothyroidism: a randomized, double-blind, crossover study. J Clin Endocrinol Metab. 2013 May;98(5):1982-90.

77. Hamilton MA, Stevenson LW, FOnarow GC, et al. Safety and Hemodynamic Effects of Intravenous Triiodothyronine in Advanced Congestive Heart Failure. American Journal of Cardiology. 1998 Feb 15;81(4)443-447.

78. Hak, EA, Pols H, Visser TJ, et al. Subclinical hypothyroidism is an independent risk factor for atherosclerosis and myocardial infarction in elderly women: The Rotterdam Study. Ann. Int. Med. 2000;132:270-278.

79. Asvold BO et al. The association between TSH within the reference range and serum lipid concentrations in a population-based study. The HUNT Study. Eur J Endocrinol. 2007 Feb;156(2):181-6.

80. Razvi S et al. The influence of age on the relationship between subclinical hypothyroidism and ischemic heart disease: a meta analysis. J Clin Endocrinol Metab. 2008

81. Iervasi, G et al. Low-T3 Syndrome, A Strong Prognostic Predictor of Death in Patients With Heart Disease Circulation. 2003;107:708

CHAPTER 9

82. Chang, C.-H.; Tsai, W.-C.; Hsu, Y.-H.; Pang, J.-H.S. Pentadecapeptide BPC 157 Enhances the Growth Hormone Receptor Expression in Tendon Fibroblasts. *Molecules* **2014**, *19*, 19066-19077.
83. D.M, Manchenko & N.Yu, Glazova & Levitskaya, Natalia & L.A, Andreeva & , KamenskiiA.A & N.F, Myasoedov. (2012). The Nootropic and Analgesic Effects of Semax

    Given via Different Routes. Neuroscience and Behavioral Physiology. 42. 264-270. 10.1007/s11055-012-9562-6.

PART 3

CHAPTER 10

84. Norman, A.W., Sunlight, season, skin pigmentation, vitamin D, and 25-hydroxyvitamin D: integral components of the vitamin D endocrine system. Am J Clin Nutr. 1998 Jun;67(6):1108-10.
85. Niacinamide therapy for joint mobility. *Conn. State Med. J.* 17:584-589, 1953
86. Niacinamide, a most neglected vitamin. 1978 Tom Spies Memorial Lecture. *J. Int. Acad. of Preventive Med.* 8:5-25,1983
87. Niacinamide improves mobility in degenerative joint disease. Abstract published in *Program of the American Association for the Advancement of Science* for its meeting in Philadelphia, May 24-30, 1986

88. https://www.semanticscholar.org/paper/Topical-nicotinamide-compared-with-clindamycin-gel-Shalita-Smith/08832c32e34761f19818af1a11c5cea211101ca7

89. Merkel RL. The use of menadione bisulfite and ascorbic acid in the treatment of nausea and vomiting of pregnancy. *American Journal of Obstetrics & Gynecology* 1952; 64:416–18.

ABOUT THE AUTHOR

Dawson Lopez is an advanced practice medical provider who specializes in weight loss and hormone therapy for both men and women. Having spent the past 35 years in the medical field, much of that time has been spent researching disease process and ways to achieve optimal health.

Instead of relying on the suggested guidelines applicable to all patients, she prefers, instead, to follow where the research leads; implementing true evidence-based practice. Bringing this research into everyday life, Dawson also gives presentations to groups of all kinds, large and small. Offering employee training on reversing obesity and improving health, Dawson helps interested businesses reduce employee absenteeism and increase productivity.

Dawson owns and provides direct patient care through Alaris Center in Tucson, Arizona, where she lives with her husband, Graciano, and their pet Bengal, Hadji.

CONTACT

To schedule a speaking engagement, please contact Dawson through

www.AlarisCenter.com

OR

email directly at

Dawson@AlarisCenter.com

To order any of the listed supplements please go to:

DawsonLopez.Metagenics.com

To contact Dawson directly:

Dawson@AlarisCenter.com